LIVES WELL LIVED GENERATIONS

Resilience, Positivity, and Purpose at Every Age

First Edition

by SKY BERGMAN

While every effort has been made to ensure the authenticity of the contributions within, any inaccuracies found are entirely unintentional. This book is a tribute to the vibrant *Lives Well Lived* film stars and to those incredible individuals and organizations dedicated to bridging generational divides, celebrating their enduring impact on our society.

ISBN 978-0-9702991-1-6
Library of Congress Control Number: 2024905648
First Edition, 2024.

For more information or to connect with Sky Bergman:

sky@skybergmanproductions.com
skybergmanproductions.com
lwlgenerations.com

Printed in the United States of America.

Magic happens when people of all ages come together. We learn, we laugh, we find our better angels. With the wonderful "Lives Well Lived – GENERATIONS," Sky Bergman inspires us to share stories and wisdom across the generations. She delivers a blueprint for going multigenerational everywhere from offices and orchestras to schools and our own homes. A book to broaden horizons, deepen understanding and lift spirits – whatever your age!

— Carl Honoré, author of *Bolder: How to Age Better and Feel Better about Aging*

"Lives Well Lived – GENERATIONS" is at once a fascinating behind-the-scenes look at filmmaker Sky Bergman's journey to create the "Lives Well Lived" documentary and an invaluable how-to-guide equipping each of us to become confident interviewers and storytellers of the elders in our lives. Intimate and pragmatic, this book reveals the power of a good question to break down barriers and create authentic, intergenerational connections. Along the way, Sky showcases the stories of more than 40 pioneering thought leaders and innovators working to bring generations together. These stories point to the possibility of a more interconnected, interdependent, and loving world and will leave you feeling motivated (and better equipped!) to craft your own life well-lived.

— Eunice Lin Nichols, Co-CEO of CoGenerate

DEDICATION

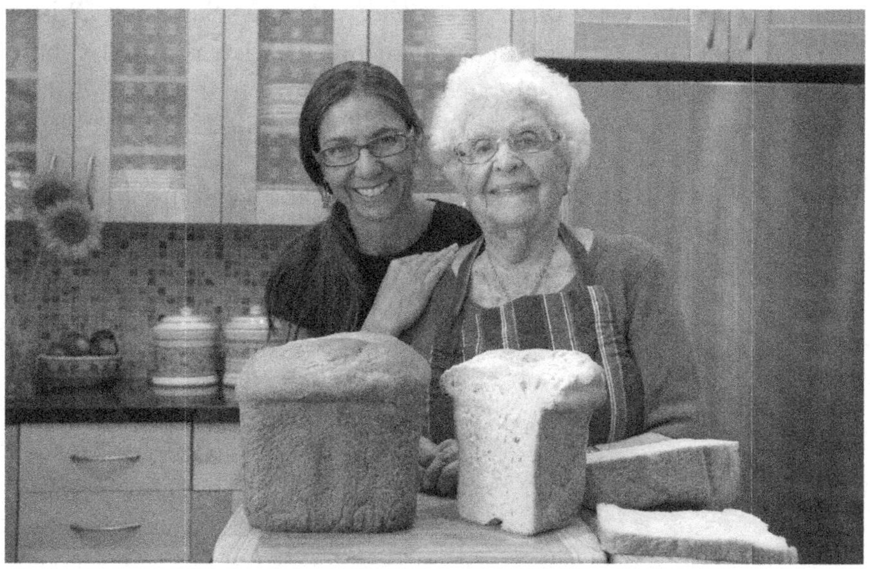

My grandmother remains my unwavering inspiration, my North Star, and my guiding light. I marveled at her resilience and her optimism. I was continually inspired by her love of life. But what I treasured the most was what my grandmother taught me. What she continues to weave into my heart, even to this day—all the wisdom, laughs, and love. I could not be the person I am today if it had not been for her. And for both of us, that is a life well lived.

She had a simple motto for her life: always be kind. At the end of my documentary film, *Lives Well Lived*, she shared, “My secret to a happy life is to live life to the fullest every day of your life. Be good to everybody you know. Do a good deed when you can and be happy.”

With deep affection, I dedicate this book, as well as the preceding film, to my beloved Grandmother—Evelyn Ricciuti, and to all the older adults featured in the film who, through their exemplary lives, teach us the profound art of living each day to its fullest.

My grandmother made the journey from Florida to California to attend a sneak preview of *Lives Well Lived* at the San Luis Obispo Film Festival. It was the best night of my life. I was able to share the film with her and twenty-seven of the forty film stars and their families. I was smiling so much that my checks hurt.

She passed away peacefully six weeks later at the remarkable age of 103. My mom says that she lived long enough to see the film on the big screen. That was her last purpose. I am forever grateful.

CONTENTS

FOREWORD

When I first watched Sky Bergman's marvelous and inspiring documentary, *Lives Well Lived*, I was so blown away I couldn't wait to write a "Worth Watching" piece about it for Next Avenue, the PBS site for people over 50.

Since then, I've been hoping Sky would turn the film into a book, sharing the lessons she learned from the 40 people featured in this film, aged 75 to 100, and explaining how the rest of us can create intergenerational projects where older people express their life lessons to younger ones.

Now she has.

This book offers terrific insights from the stars of the film, mixed with humor and grace as well as personal triumphs and tragedies to help us lead our best lives as we age.

Sky also includes essential advice from people running pioneering programs that are bringing generations together—from CoGenerate to Generations United to Eldera to the Eisner Intergenerational Music Program to Champions of Caring—and from leaders of initiatives like the Modern Elder Academy to the advocates dedicated to erasing ageism at Changing the Narrative.

Reading their thoughtful recommendations and then putting them into action, I believe, will help make great strides in fostering much needed intergenerational relationships.

This book also demonstrates how much older and younger people have in common and why the idea of intergenerational conflict is pernicious, if not bogus.

Sky Bergman began her walk down the path that led to this book by chatting with her grandmother, Evelyn, watching her work out at the gym at age 99 and spending time together making memories and delicious food in the kitchen.

These conversations and moments blossomed into the *Lives Well Lived* documentary where dozens of other older adults with 3,000 years of collective life experience, told Sky about their exceptional life stories.

This book now takes the idea further by showing readers what Sky calls the four common threads constituting a fulfilling life. Then, she provides practical tips about how to weave those threads into your life by finding purpose and support groups, learning how to enjoy a positive outlook, becoming resilient and creating intergenerational projects. She also offers important questions to ask yourself to help you along this journey.

One of my favorite themes of this book is that retirement can now be a new chapter filled with possibilities. I've found that to be true personally in my 'unretirement' and have written about this in "The View From Unretirement" column on MarketWatch.

In her own life, Sky Bergman took an unexpected leap, retiring from 30 years of teaching photography to college students and embarking on her new chapters as a filmmaker, author and intergenerational project leader.

After reading this book, I think you'll be very glad she did.

Richard Eisenberg
"The View From Unretirement" columnist, MarketWatch and former Managing Editor of Next Avenue

INTRODUCTION

For tens of thousands of years, humans have looked to the older adults in their lives for wisdom and experience on how to survive and thrive in a world full of challenges. From the Native American Indians to the Australian Aborigines, verbal stories were the how-to guides that were handed down from generation to generation.

As the 21st Century began, the advent of technology and the internet meant that—overnight—information was everywhere. Almost, in the blink of an eye, our world turned its back on our elders as the source of wisdom and experience. In fact, the last hundred years is the first time we have looked to anyone other than our elders for advice. Lest we forget, knowledge isn't wisdom and information is not experience.

Regardless of race, gender, sexual orientation, ability, or socioeconomic status, the one thing we have in common is that we age every day. Yet we are constantly bombarded by negative stereotypes of aging. The "graying of America" is no longer a futuristic prediction: the Beatles appeared on *The Ed Sullivan Show* sixty years ago and baby boomers are turning 80.

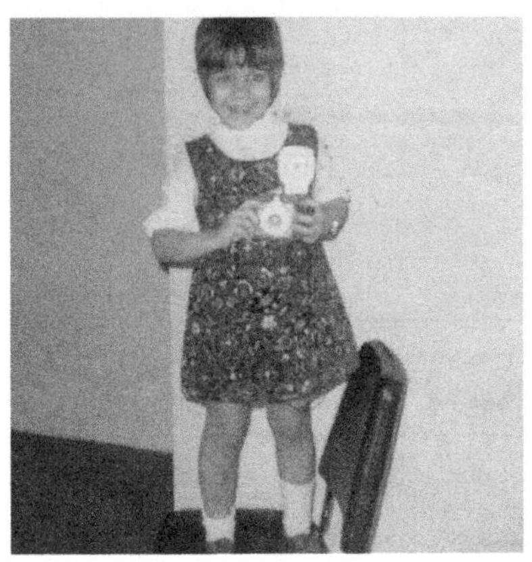

As I was approaching my 50th year and starting to reflect on my own life, I began a quest to search for other people who were living life to the limits and could be positive role models for aging.

My grandmother, Evelyn, quite by serendipitous accident, became the first star of my documentary film, *Lives Well Lived.* We spent a lot of time together—often in the kitchen cooking together. It was here that she passed on wisdom from her life, and at the same time inspired the journey that led to the film and this book. I've experienced the most wonderful and deeply personal journey over the last couple of years, and I want to share my experience with you. I have always believed that the more personal the story, the more universal.

Along with my grandmother, I have been fortunate to document the life experiences of dozens of elders. While creating the *Lives Well Lived* film, I interviewed people aged 75-100 with a collective life experience of 3000 years. The stories they shared have been heartwarming, joyful and heart-rending. Their lives are both deep in lessons and broad in scope. In a sense, they are like a tapestry where the colors of the threads illustrate their history of rich and purposeful lives.

The film interviewees opened the vault on their journey into aging through family histories, personal triumphs and tragedies, loves and losses—seeing the best and worst of humanity along the way. Their stories are about perseverance, the human spirit, and staying positive during great personal and historic challenges. Their stories will make you laugh and cry, but ultimately, I hope they will inspire you.

As a result of my experience, I've seen patterns and trends that have led me to understand what contributes to a life well lived, both from the perspective of the person who lived it and from those who were part of it. As the documentary film *Lives Well Lived* told the stories of the individuals, this book aims to share the patterns and themes to inform you and others about the power of positive aging. Perhaps it will help you to seek out the important people in your life to understand their journey, or to inspire you on your own journey to a life well lived.

Along the way, you will meet…

- 78-year-old former civil rights activist who now teaches Afro-Haitian dance.
- an 80-year-old Latino-Filipino educator who teaches English as a second language and who is six units away from earning her Ph.D.
- 92-year-old retired doctor who wakes up early every morning to make mozzarella for his daughter's delicatessen.
- 95-year-old who lived through the Japanese Internment.

What can we learn from their stories? The *Lives Well Lived* film captured the images, ideas, and ideals of those who are proving that aging is something to cherish, that retirement doesn't mean you retire from life, and that growing older doesn't mean growing silent. These are the people teaching a growing population of men and women how to age with dignity, grace, energy, and purpose. In the following chapters, we will explore each of the four common threads that I observed along my journey with the film of what constituted a fulfilling, meaningful life:

- **Having a sense of purpose at every age**
- **Building a strong support network, whether that is family or friends**
- **Enjoying a positive outlook on life**
- **Being resilient**

Of course, while others may comment that we are ultimately the harshest critics of our lives—what we are proud of and what we regret, one thing is certain: no one person's life could answer this question. It is my belief that we need many people, and many lives, to see patterns and themes around what constitutes a good life.

When was the last time that you sat down with an older adult and engaged in a meaningful conversation? Our modern world differs from those of our distant ancestors sitting around the campfire sharing stories and wisdom. I was lucky; I grew up in an Italian household with four generations around the dinner table where the stories, wisdom, and knowledge would flow. Picture this: the aroma of Grandma's lasagna wafting in the air, the sound of plates clinking and gesturing of hands as the stories got louder and more elaborate as the meal went on. When the fruit and nuts came out, that was when the stories were at their best. My childhood was filled with intergenerational connection to older adults, and that played such an important role in my development and outlook on life.

As we wind through this journey together, I will give you the structure to interview and connect with an older adult in your life. I also encourage organizational leaders and educators to return to the campfire, and to explore the potential for intergenerational connections where research continues to show the benefits of a diverse, age-inclusive world. In further chapters, I will provide you with methods that you can use to bring an intergenerational project to your community, educational institution, corporation, or even to your own family.

I will introduce you to leading experts in the field and people who are doing inspiring intergenerational work. I have asked them to answer the questions, "What is the value of intergenerational programs? What positive outcomes do you see achieved through intergenerational programs?" I hope to leave you inspired by the work of a variety of organizations that are connecting generations in innovative and exciting ways.

You don't have to be a celebrity or impact the lives of millions to have lived a life well lived. The scale of your fame has nothing to do with it. The truth is that everyone has an impact by the way they live, and what seems to matter most is having a purpose, being supported by others, keeping positive, and being resilient.

My lofty goal is to inspire you on your own journey toward a life well lived, to take you on a voyage thousands of years in the living.

We have a generation of older adults who've lived through the toughest of times, and now a generation is coming of age during the toughest of times. If we can find our common ground by creating intergenerational connections—especially in times of social unrest and isolation—we can help one another create a better tomorrow. So let us dive in and see what makes a life well lived and how we can all benefit by connecting generations. For tens of thousands of years, humans have looked to the older adults in their lives for wisdom and experience on how to survive and thrive in a world full of challenges. From the Native American Indians to the Australian Aborigines, verbal stories were the how-to guides that were handed down from generation to generation.

SECTION ONE

INSPIRATION

MY PURPOSE FOR FILMING LIVES WELL LIVED AND WRITING GENERATIONS

As I was approaching my 50th birthday, my grandmother was also approaching a major birthday milestone. She was about to celebrate 100 trips around the sun. I will feel incredibly fortunate if I can achieve that milestone, but even more important, I look forward to using the second half of my life to inspire others and be a role model, just as my grandmother, Evelyn, did for me.

At the time, I noticed a disconnect between what I was learning through my grandmother's example of how to age well and what the media was portraying. Most movies, and indeed commercial advertising, were showing the negative aspects of aging. Advertising promoted anti-aging creams and potions and the need to look younger; while my grandmother was busy working out at the gym and reveling in her older age. I wasn't seeing the positive aspects of aging that were so visibly inspiring to me in my grandmother. I felt an urge to see more positive stories and messages. Back then, the idea of a documentary film wasn't even a twinkle in my eye, but that first thought would eventually morph into a concept, and then into the film, and then, my passion.

My grandmother's cooking…

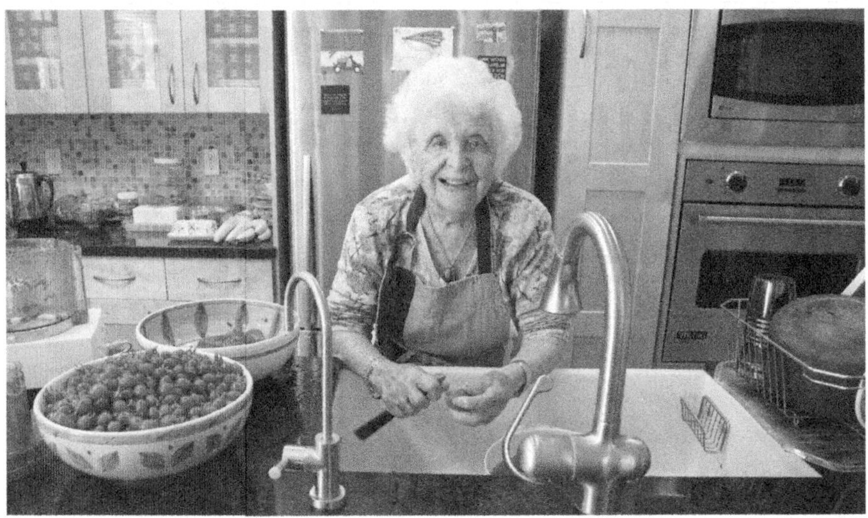

My first foray into the world of filmmaking began when my grandmother came out to visit me for the first time, traveling from Florida to California. She was 96 years old, and we would go to the farmer's market on Thursday night, and then Friday, we would cook all day. Grandma would make all these wonderful dishes that we would then freeze. Like any Italian grandmother, she was worried that I would not have enough to eat. By the time she left, my freezer was filled to the brim with delicious food.

Along the way, I realized something. Yes, my grandmother was an amazing cook—but this was also her way of showing love. Being in the kitchen together was a time when we really connected, as she would share wonderful stories while we cooked together. I realized at that time that I didn't have any of her recipes written down. Even if I did try to document them, I couldn't really quantify the recipes because, like many people who've been cooking all their lives, each recipe was more a matter of the love that my grandmother put into it. You know the story, a 'handful of this,' and a 'spoonful of that,' with a little pinch of happiness thrown in.

As a result, I decided to record, not just the recipe itself, but the act of my grandmother making the food, her gestures, the sound of her voice, the little things that cannot be captured in a written recipe or photograph. Up to that point, I had been a still photographer, but my desire to capture her nuances pushed my creative process into my first foray into the world of filmmaking. The creation of a little series that I called Cucina Nonna (Italian for 'Grandma's Kitchen') was born.

It was all about documenting this wonderful time with my grandmother cooking in the kitchen, and it also became my first adventure into doing anything with film or video. Although I didn't realize it at the time, this was the beginning of my passion for documenting someone's story on film. Looking back, this idea (or purpose) had an early beginning. As a youngster, I would put the tape recorder on the table during Sunday dinners and, being an Italian household, we would talk for hours. Officially collecting somebody's story—in terms of the moving image—really started with those videos of my grandmother cooking.

One day, at the gym…

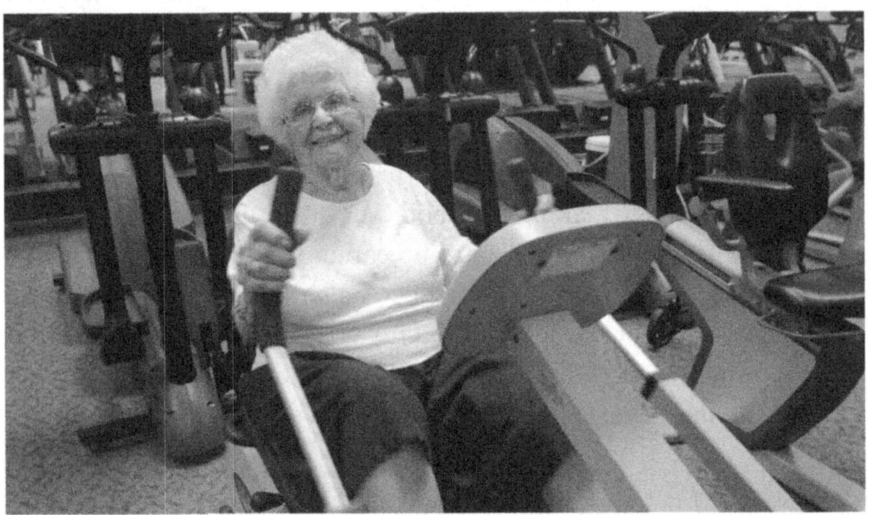

When I visited my grandmother for her hundredth birthday, I filmed her exercising because I thought, *nobody is going to believe that, at almost a hundred, my grandma is working out at the gym*. Those precious moments in the gym, with her on the exercise bike, were really the beginning of the *Lives Well Lived* film.

I remember distinctly the moment when, as a throwaway comment, I asked her, "Hey, Grandma, can you give me some words of wisdom?"

Let's picture that moment together.

We're in a local gym, like *any* local gym. There is equipment around, a slight smell of perspiration in the air. The click and clack of weights being picked up and set down. The whir of fans in the ceiling. The hum of bikes and rowing machines. There is Evelyn, a ninety-nine-year-old, and by far the oldest person in the gym. She is on an exercise bike, and while she is pedaling, she looks at me and replies, "Live life to the limits. Be kind."

Right then and there, I had the epiphany. The light bulb went off. I thought, *this is what I'm meant to be doing, right here and right now.* There I was, with my beautiful and wise grandmother who was about to turn 100 in two days. She has just shared those simple, yet powerful, words of wisdom.

At that moment, I felt a deep and moving desire to go out and find other people like my grandmother who are also living amazing lives. I wanted to find people who would be positive role models of age, aging and life, people who could show me and others, what I was not seeing in the media. These were people who had lived, and were living, a life of meaning and purpose.

The intergenerational project begins...

When I first began the project, I really wanted to interview and speak with everyday people, ordinary people. I wanted those who were watching the film and reading the interviews to be reminded of somebody who could be in their family or even themselves. I wanted them to connect. I just started interviewing people, without having any idea of what I was going to do with all these interviews.

To find everyday people, I enlisted the help of my friends, family and former students by sending an email to roughly a thousand people with a link to the video of my grandmother at the gym asking, "If you have somebody in your life that's as much an inspiration as my grandmother is to me, please nominate them for this project." Soon after, I was inundated with heartwarming nominations from across the country, and overwhelmed by the breadth of different kinds of people with varied life experiences.

I felt it was important to start with a good list of questions that I would ask each participant in the project, so I took my time planning and developing the questions over a six-month period. As a professor at a university, I reached out to my colleagues in the Psychology and

Social Sciences department. I asked them, "If you were working on a project like this, interviewing people aged 75-100, what questions would you ask?"

The twenty questions I crafted formed the initial framework for the interviews, designed to be open-ended and flexible, allowing for many tangents along the way. I wanted the questions to be open-ended to leave room to elicit meaningful responses about the participants' life experiences and their history. This approach fostered a space where people felt comfortable sharing their life's journey and delving into aspects of their personal history.

I embarked on the project, questions in hand, doing several interviews and putting together a few little five-minute snapshot videos, thinking I might do a web series. I wasn't sure what the end result would be, but what I did know was that I was driven to meet these people and to collect their stories. My belief is that everyone has an interesting story to share, if we just take the time to listen.

I've spoken about the serendipity of asking my grandmother for her advice. Another pivotal moment on my journey was when I interviewed Marion Wolff.

Marion Wolff's story of hope and resilience...

Marion Wolff was born in Berlin, Germany in 1930. With the arrival of the Nazi persecution of Jews, she fled with her parents to Vienna, Austria in 1936, only to experience the full might of Hitler's wrath after the infamous 'Night of Broken Glass' in 1938. Very soon after, at the age eight, Marion left Vienna for England on the first experimental Kindertransport. The Kindertransport was a remarkable rescue mission that took place on the eve of World War II. Initiated in 1938, it was a humanitarian program that saved approximately 10,000 predominantly Jewish children from Nazi-occupied territories. Her plight, along with 10,000 other unaccompanied Jewish children without their parents, was captured by the Hearst Corporation's "News of the Day" footage where Marion made an unwitting appearance as she disembarked the ship into the arms of a Quaker foster family.

During our interview, Marion had an item to show me. It is a moment that will live with me forever. You see, Marion still had the cardboard number given to her in Austria that she wore around her neck at the age of eight years old to identify her on her journey to freedom from Austria to her new life in the UK. I still get chills even writing these words about that little cardboard number. That moment really made me consider my own life. *What was I doing when I was eight years old? What was I going through?*

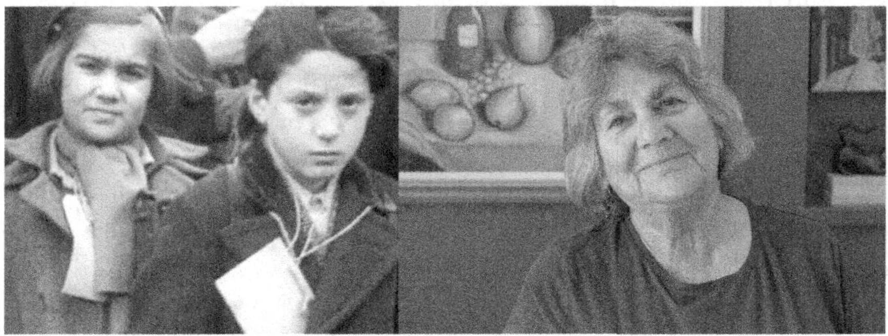

Left: Marion Wolff at age 8 during her Kindertransport from Vienna, Austria. Right: Marion Wolff, age 84

Here was somebody who lived this moment in time, a moment that has become ingrained in our collective consciousness. She was there. It really shifted my view on what this project was all about. In the beginning, I was just thinking I was going to collect the words of wisdom of wonderful older adults. Instead, it morphed into a journey of collecting their stories of resilience and all the experiences they had to overcome.

Following a passion...

My collection of stories was too important to think small. These narratives were profoundly impactful, deserving more than just brief video segments. I realized it would be even more powerful to weave the stories into a cohesive, full-length documentary to hopefully expose their narratives to a wider and larger audience.

I always joke about the fact that I don't know why I thought I could just up and make a film. I'd never created a film before, but somehow it just felt like the right thing to do. I have always been one of those people that have followed my passion and my intuition. That little voice in my head that says, *you may not know exactly why you're doing this right at this moment, but this is the right thing to be doing.* For me, it is really important that I've just followed my passion wherever that's led me.

Now, making a film is quite a challenge. Anyone who decides on a purpose or a goal will run into challenges. Many times during the course of making the film, I thought, *what the heck am I doing? I've never done this before.* I had no idea how to create or finance a film. But even though I was a novice and didn't have a hefty bank account, I never let these obstacles get in the way of pursuing what I become truly passionate about. It was this deep-rooted passion, and clear purpose, that fueled my determination to make it happen.

Throughout my life, I have always believed that if you are driven to accomplish something, with a lot of tenacity and resilience, you can make just about anything happen.

I have always been of the mindset to embrace opportunities with a 'why not?' attitude, rather than obstructing them with doubts by asking 'why?'. I follow my heart and keep my mind open to ideas that might sound a little crazy. The worst thing that could happen is I fall flat and fail, but the potential reward of following what might seem like a crazy dream is creating something truly extraordinary.

Financing the film…

My first stumbling block in producing a film was the financing. As a university professor, my initial thought was to apply for grants to fund the project, but I was rejected for all but one small grant that would barely cover much more than a few students to assist. I realized that I would have to get creative and bootstrap the project myself. My solution: I had several unused rooms in my house, so I decided to list them on Airbnb. That was how I raised the funds to creatively finance the film by renting rooms in my house over a number of years. I have never let money be an obstacle, the reason why I did or didn't do something. Sometimes, you have to think outside the box to make things happen.

I will admit that I was in way above my head, having never created a film before. At the university where I teach, we have a motto, "Learn by Doing." I was a living, breathing example of that principle. Beyond securing funding, I faced a substantial learning curve regarding the overall filmmaking process. It was quite a daunting task, but I am not afraid to ask for help and to admit my lack of expertise in certain areas. I frequently visited the Apple store, engaging with the experts there for advice on editing and filmmaking techniques. I also reached out to other filmmakers and would say, "Wow, I love what you're doing, and I'd love to connect with you and hear more about your process." I think that many of us have a fear of saying we don't know what we're doing, showing our cards, and saying, "I'm really a novice at this, and I would love to have your help." When you do open yourself up, people want to help, especially if you talk about what it is that you admire in them. Most people want to give back in some way. I've found that just by being humble and saying, "I don't understand. I don't know. But you're doing something that I'd love to be doing, and can I be a fly on the wall?" Or, "Can I take you out for coffee and connect with you, and just share some ideas?"

Finding your tribe...

Through this process, I have learned the power of surrounding myself with people who excel in the areas one aspires to and acknowledging that a collaborative effort is essential. So, I assembled a team of talented individuals to assist with sound, editing, and research, ensuring a supportive environment for the creation of the film. Think about all the credits at the end of any film. It takes a literal village of collective effort to tackle a project of this scale. Through this collective endeavor, there is no loss, only gain, and it results in the work shining even more brilliantly. It brings to mind a quote I came across years ago: "A candle doesn't diminish its own radiance when it ignites another candle."

There were certainly moments during that where I thought, *is this just pure folly?* I think we all have doubts at times. I would get up at 4 a.m. and start editing before teaching my classes at the university. Some mornings, I would think, 7But my answer was quite clear: a deep love of my grandmother, and all the people that I interviewed, kept me focused. In those moments of doubt, I would hear my inner voice reminding me that I needed to get their stories of resilience, hope, and strength out in the world. This strong sense of purpose and passion got me through, over, and around some very tough moments.

All you need is one *YES!*

It reminded me of another time where I had to defy the odds. As a relatively young Master of Fine Arts graduate in search of a teaching job, I applied to more than 300 jobs before landing my teaching position. I kept all the rejection letters for years as a poignant reminder that all it takes is one acceptance. All it takes is one, 'yes,' one person to believe in you!

Needless to say, when you're going through all the rejections, it can sometimes be quite difficult to keep your chin up and push on through. Even during our film festival run, there was one day when I received six email rejections in a row, and I was totally disheartened. Again, I reminded myself that one acceptance makes all the difference in the world, one person to say, “Wow, I love that, and I want to help you distribute it.” You really have to believe in what you’re doing, and my method, when faced with those moments, certainly begins with a reminder of purpose.

I also walk or do yoga to clear my head, think about ideas, and about how I can change the narrative. Just getting away from the computer and looking at things from a different vantage point, different scenery, and doing something physical, like walking and breathing fresh air, makes all the difference. One of the great lessons that I learned from the people in the film is to live in the moment; if I’m getting upset that something’s not happening, I’m not really living in the moment.

The art of listening…

Few of us have the luxury of time to simply listen to people. I’ve had the good fortune to take time to listen to the forty people from my film with a collective life experience of 3,000 years! I was looking for people who could be positive role models with a diverse background. While I went looking for diversity, I ended up finding commonality. No matter where these people came from, their lives reflected the similar themes. Maybe they faced different challenges, but they came to the same conclusions about what was important to them. We have overlying commonalities no matter who we are and where we have come from; it’s just about being human. We need to have a sense of purpose and a sense of connection. No matter what you’ve been through, those are still the core elements of what it takes to really feel as if you’ve had a meaningful life.

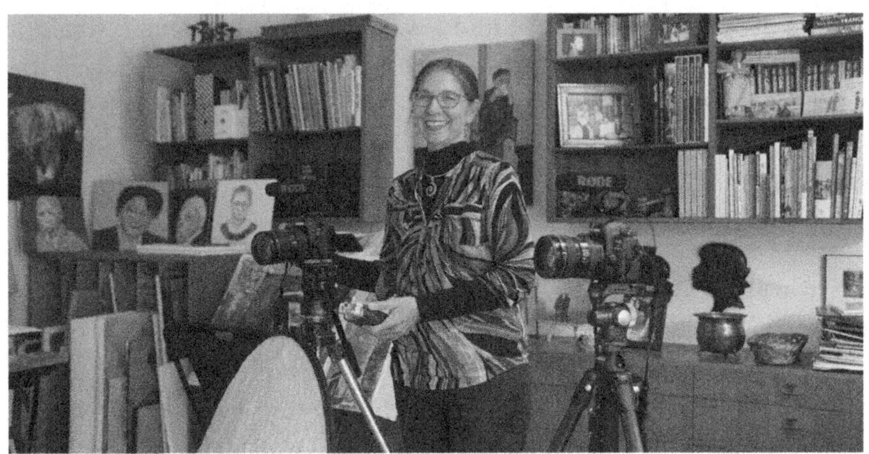

Mind you, it's not just about looking back. These themes can help someone who wants to live a meaningful, well-lived life. It is about continuing to look forward and creating a future. Everyone featured in the film was continuing to look forward. I've gained a wealth of wisdom from listening to their journeys, understanding their methods, and learning what has been effective for them. Now, I'm eager to pass on these insights to you.

FIND YOUR PURPOSE

"I look forward to the next hour, the next day, and no plans. I take what comes and absorb it as much as I can, mentally, physically, emotionally, visually, audibly. I drink it up."

— Wachtang 'Botso' Korisheli, *Lives Well Lived* film star, age 93

Looking forward to the future is, of course, a purpose in and of itself. If we have no purpose, we cannot conceive of, let alone, begin to create a future since there is no reason for us to do so. Therefore, purpose, in my mind is both a precursor *to* and creator *of* the future.

I'd like you to imagine this scene. One bright, warm and sunny morning, you look out of your window and gaze up at a mountaintop in the distance. You decide to take a walk to the top of that mountain and begin to prepare what you will need for the walk. You get food and water, along with some tools and other useful items that will help you on the journey. You get dressed in some comfortable walking clothes and shoes. You set out on the path.

Life is very much like walking a path to the top of a mountain. All of us find something we love doing, and we set our goals, and work toward them. At times, we run into challenges and barriers that we have to overcome in order to reach those goals. At certain moments, we take stock of what we have achieved. Sometimes, we may choose a different path or join up with someone who walks the path with us. There might be moments when we stop to take a breath and admire the view. Sometimes the trail is flat and easy to travel; at other times, it is rocky and hilly, and it takes the wind out of our sails. Overcoming a challenge can bring great joy.

I feel the best way to describe a purpose or goal is the mountaintop itself. The mountain peak is what we are trying to achieve in our life—either short or long term. This goal might be to complete our schooling and gain enough knowledge to transition to a professional career. It might be to find a life partner, get married, and start the next generation. Or, perhaps it is to gradually gain experience and wisdom, advancing in our careers so we can set ourselves up for a secure retirement.

However, retirement often marks a significant transition in life, where many individuals face the challenge of redefining their sense of purpose. For a large part of our lives, our identities are closely intertwined with our careers. In social settings, when asked about what we do, our professions often define the response, thus becoming a core part of our self-identity. This deep association can lead to a sense of loss or emptiness when we step away from our careers upon retiring.

Overcoming this challenge involves a deliberate shift in perspective and a journey of self-discovery. Retirement can be seen not as an end, but as a new chapter full of possibilities. It's an opportunity to explore interests that were sidelined due to career commitments or to discover new passions. Engaging in volunteer work, pursuing hobbies, or even learning new skills can instill a renewed sense of purpose.

Lucky Louie Tedone continued making mozzarella for his daughter's delicatessen when he was 96, as he had done for many years. This was despite him having a busy and successful working life as a pediatrician for over fifty years. His purpose had changed over his life from caring for young children to making those delicious round balls of creamy dairy goodness in order to support his daughter's business. Lou said during our interview that he felt he got his purpose and philosophy from his parents.

"My parents worked very hard in the store since there were no other employees, never had a day off and never complained about it. They were so proud that they were able to provide a decent living, that there was food on the table. I developed that philosophy: that you do the best you can, do your job, and work hard."

For Marion and Paul Wolff, talking about their experiences in the Holocaust fueled their desire to ensure future generations would not repeat the mistakes of those terrible times. Marion shared their purpose in our discussions:

"We consciously make an effort to speak at local schools because we feel an obligation to tell our story. We are not going to be here forever, and then, how truthfully will our story be told?"

Marion and Paul were concerned about who was going to be able to tell this history with reality and truth once they were gone. We all know history can be like 'Chinese whispers' when it passes from the originator through other voices. Marion's view is one that I share—If you want to know the reality about some situation or event, you are better to hear it from the people who've gone through it rather than from a history book.

Rose expressed her purpose in teaching English as a second language to students. Learning English had been an important steppingstone in her life, so she wanted to give something back.

"I have compassion for the students that I work with because I know firsthand how difficult it is for them to learn a second language. So, I volunteer at the high school every morning."

Time and again, interview after inspiring interview, I saw this theme of giving back, passing on, returning the favor, or sharing experience as fuel for the fire of purpose. Purpose was there to drive them on, through thick and thin. This sentiment was shared when I spoke to those influenced by these purposeful individuals. When children, friends or colleagues observed that a person was fueled by a broader purpose, it was appreciated by those receiving it without exception. Humans, therefore, seem to notice when another person is driven by purpose, whether it is a passion to give back, or pay forward, or help others. We respond with warmth, joy, and thankfulness for that individual's presence on this little blue marble we call Earth.

One of the interesting things I've noticed in the individuals I spoke with is that having a purpose served to help them create a future. This future may have only existed in the mind of the individual. Nevertheless, it was real to them and as the majority I spoke with were in their seventies, eighties, and nineties, it did contribute anecdotally to a long life for them. But this anecdotal evidence has been backed by significant scientific research. Across many studies, scientists and doctors have proven that people with a purpose tend to live longer and healthier lives.

Purpose provides an outward focus and takes the attention of the individual off themselves and onto the task or purpose where they have chosen to direct their efforts, time and attention. I have no doubt in my mind that Lou lived longer because he made mozzarella. I have no doubt that Paul—in his nineties and currently working on a presentation for an upcoming event—is contributing to this day because of his deep desire to share his Holocaust experiences.

Specific research into retirement has suggested that those who leave work and don't replace that purpose with something else—a sport, volunteering, gardening, or some other activity—tend to die earlier than those who continue to lead purposeful lives beyond their income-earning or working lives.

For me, personally, after a thirty-year university career teaching photography, I decided to retire from teaching. My colleagues asked me, "Why are you retiring so young when you are at the top of your game?" I realized that I had fulfilled my teaching career and decided to look through a different creative lens: filmmaking. I was lucky enough to be able to walk away and re-invent myself at 56 years old.

I have choices about what my sense of purpose will be. I believe that no matter which decade of age, whether it is 20, 40, 60, 80, or beyond, we all need to find our sense of purpose, the drive that keeps us going, that feeds our curiosity. I also believe that our sense of purpose can change over time depending on our life circumstances. For me, creating a film about older adults changed mine.

For my dad, a practicing geriatric physician, having and surviving two strokes reinvigorated his sense of purpose. The first stroke, when he was in his forties, required a very experimental brain surgery. It took him a year to recuperate, but he resumed working as soon as he could. His second stroke, at 69, left him with one side of his body weakened enough to require being mostly in a wheelchair, but able to walk short distances with a walker. He lost the ability to do many of the things he loved, such as playing the guitar and practicing archery. The one thing he could still do well, however, was practice medicine. His perseverance has made him a role model for his patients. When I asked him why he continued treating patients, he explained that he did so out of his sense of purpose, his passion, and the desire to be productive. Despite even greater challenges, my dad continued his medical practice until his passing, just shy of 80 years old.

"He who has a why to live can bear almost any how."

— Friedrich Nietzsche

That quote underscores the significant impact that a strong sense of purpose, or a 'why,' has on an individual's life. It conveys the idea that understanding one's purpose, or reasons for living, equips a person with the strength to withstand and triumph over numerous challenges and hardships. This profound insight, encapsulated in a single sentence, speaks volumes about the concepts of resilience, motivation, and the essence of the human experience.

Many times in life, we just go on day to day, so busy with our lives that we don't have that moment to pause and really think about what we are doing, what we are grateful for, and what feeds our soul. Are you able to really look at your life and find your true sense of purpose and happiness in the world? How will you redefine your life and your sense of purpose? If and when you do, you may find that committing to that purpose is a vital ingredient of a life well lived.

Steps to finding your own purpose...

Now that we've heard from some of the stars of our documentary, it's time to turn the lens inward. Are you clear about your life's purpose, or do you find yourself in a state of uncertainty or transition? The term 'purposeful' resonates with intention and direction, so let's begin by looking ahead. I encourage you to ponder over these three reflective questions:

- *What future do you imagine for yourself?*
- *What accomplishments do you aspire to achieve?*
- *How do you wish to make a difference and who do you want to impact?*

These questions are not just introspective exercises; they serve to either reaffirm your existing, motivating purpose or to aid in uncovering a path that shapes your future. As I've learned from my interviews, knowing your purpose and crafting a future around it, is not just fulfilling—it's also life-enhancing.

This journey can include engaging in volunteer activities, indulging in hobbies, or acquiring new skills, all of which can reignite a sense of purpose. Building stronger relationships with family and friends and contributing to the community in impactful ways are also part of this journey. Redefining your purpose beyond just a professional identity can lead to a life that is not only fulfilling but also rich in personal growth and new experiences.

SUPPORT

"The secret to a happy life is having good friends who support you; I know this has been incredibly important in my own life!"

— Barbara Gesino, *Lives Well Lived* film star, age 75

In the diverse stories shared throughout the documentary interviews, a resounding theme emerged, reminiscent of the timeless adage, "It takes a village to raise a child." This ancient wisdom, underscoring the quintessence of communal support and interconnectedness, has been a cornerstone of human civilization. It harkens back to our ancestral roots when families were the nucleus for growth, sharing of wisdom, and collective flourishing.

Our lives are enriched by the strength and presence of others, whether through supporting our goals or simply by being there. This means offering non-judgmental, supportive companionship, creating a robust foundation for life's journey. Each interviewee spoke of family and friends who stood by them in joy and adversity, providing a listening ear or a helping hand when needed.

A simple example of this that I experienced myself involved Lucky Louie. Over the years, Lou became a close friend. It was a pleasure to share his story and his life experiences. One day, I was due to go and meet Lou, but I was feeling under the weather. Since Lou was in his nineties, I didn't want to bring illness into his home, so I called and gave my apologies. Soon after, fresh homemade chicken soup mysteriously appeared on my doorstep. Of course, it was from Lou.

At 96, he made the effort to cook me a soup and deliver it. It was true to his generous personality and his interest in cooking good food for others. He wanted to help ensure I was okay and looked after. I was humbled by this beautiful gesture from Lou, and it is a moment I will treasure for as long as I live. I hope I can pass on similar gestures to family and friends around me as I continue my quest for my own life well lived.

That experience (as with so many others in my life) has proven the idea that support is a critical element of our lives. It reaffirmed my belief that it would be impossible to have a life well lived unless it involved the support, encouragement, love, and attention of others around us. And indeed, where we provide that same support and love to others around us, it becomes both the fuel in our engines and—if you'll pardon the gooey cliche—the wind beneath our wings.

"Alone we can do so little; together, we can do so much."

— Helen Keller

When I was in my forties, I noticed that when illness or misadventure entered the lives of our friends, it was most often our female friends that mobilized to support us. I came to the startling realization that I didn't have anywhere near enough friends in my life. I'd thrown myself into my career and, as many career-oriented people do, had let that work and mission contribute to an unbalanced life and social network. I thought, I *have lots of work associates but not enough personal connections.* I decided to be proactive and do something to change that. It had to be something that was easy enough for me to add to my busy life, so I came up with the idea of a monthly women's potluck dinner. Over the course of a decade, I have shared many beautiful evenings with women of all ages as a result. Every month, there are new women that show up at my doorstep. I have met so many amazing people that I would never have bonded with otherwise. My friend network is now brimming and full. I have a much broader and deeper support system around me than I would have if I'd continued to place a more unbalanced emphasis on work rather than the whole of life, all from the simple act of breaking bread together.

There have been numerous studies that have proven that having friends is as important as diet and exercise for living longer. Social connection is essential throughout a person's lifespan. In fact, the longest running study on happiness by Dr. Robert Waldinger, a professor of psychiatry at Harvard Medical School and author of *The Good Life*, revealed that the number one key to living longer is good relationships. (Gostick, 2023)

Echoing this sentiment, the narratives captured in the film vividly illustrated the diverse forms and faces of support that anchor our lives. Whether it was the enduring bond of a couple in a longstanding union, the unwavering support of family, or the invaluable presence of friends, these relationships stood as lighthouses guiding us through life's tempests. In every story, the underlying motif was clear: the network of support, be it through a spouse, family, or friends, is a treasure beyond measure, a cornerstone in the architecture of a life well lived.

Building your support network…

Do you have a good support network of friends, family, and groups to which you belong?

It was clear during this project that a support network was incredibly important to the people I interviewed. I'm not talking about this being one way, a selfish exercise where these people leaned on others to help them fulfill their own goals. It was most definitely a two-way street.

Those I interviewed were equally supportive of the people in their networks. What this meant was they spent their lives depositing 'value' into their group, into a communal well of good works, supportive deeds, and helpful actions. When they really needed that group, it was returned with interest. My interviewees noticed the value of not feeling lonely; they noticed the value of having someone to care for, and someone who would care for them in return.

What types of support networks can you create in your life?

The first stop on your journey will no doubt be obvious—as it was for many of the interviewees. Family and friends form the backbone of support for many. This was the same for my grandmother—and yet, she also had a large network of contacts outside of the family—as evidenced by the more than eighty people who attended her 100th birthday party. This certainly was a testament to her strong connections in her community.

Finding groups of people with whom you can interact and potentially form friendships involves exploring various avenues and opportunities that align with your interests, lifestyle, and values. Remember, the key to forming friendships is not about where you meet people, but about being open, approachable, and willing to invest time in building relationships. You might even decide to open your home and have a big dinner party once a month. It does not have to be a heavy lift, perhaps simply a potluck or a book club at your house. Make it something that sparks joy and opens a space for friendships and connections that you can count on in your life.

Source:

Gostick, Adrian. Harvard Research Reveals The #1 Key To Living Longer And Happier. Forbes.com. August 15, 2023. https://bit.ly/49ETwgS

POSITIVITY AND ATTITUDE

"When I wake up in the morning, I expect something good to happen. I don't know exactly what it would be, and sometimes it's postponed until the next day, or the day after. But inevitably, there's something wonderful that will happen."

— Rachael Winn Yon, *Lives Well Lived* film star, age 78

I adore photography. It is a vocation and profession for me. In photography, you literally spend your time looking through a small viewfinder, aiming to find the perfect 'framing'—as in a subject framed by the edges of the viewfinder. It might be a person's face, or a landscape, or a stormy sky. And this term— 'framing'—or more accurately REFRAMING, came to mind so often in my interviews and discussions. It was such a powerful theme in the lives of all my interviewees that it had to become part of this book. Each of these individuals showed an ability to reframe experiences—especially those sad, tough or downright dire moments—and to find or reframe them in a positive light. It certainly speaks to another theme that I noticed amongst these individuals, which I will speak of later. That theme is resilience.

How do we reframe an event to look on it as a positive moment rather than a negative experience?

Lucky Louie is once again a lovely example of positivity. He told me a story that exemplifies his nickname:

He borrowed a friend's car to drive a fairly long trip to a conference in the Bay Area and he had an accident. But they were so lucky because the car still drove. Then the tire blew out, and they were so lucky because they had a spare tire. Then they got up to San Francisco, and the conference he was supposed to go to was cancelled. He said, "Oh, we're so lucky. We get to spend the day in San Francisco."

At times, all of us will need an attitude adjustment, a moment to stand back and look at what is happening at that time and reframe how we remember it. Perhaps this is merely a self-protective mechanism, but according to a Mayo Clinic study (Mayo Clinic, 2023), people that look at life as the glass as half full rather than half empty live a longer life.

In their research, the Mayo Clinic asserts that, "It's unclear why people who engage in positive thinking experience these health benefits. One theory is that having a positive outlook enables you to cope better with stressful situations which reduces the harmful health effects of stress on your body."

Their research also suggests that positive and optimistic people tend to lead healthier lifestyles through diet and physical activity. They tend to avoid smoking and drinking alcohol in excess. And they learn the habit of turning negative thinking into positive thinking through time and practice.

The power of positive thinking lies in its ability to transform our perspective, influencing our emotional, psychological, and physical well-being. It's a tool that empowers individuals to face life's challenges with resilience and hope, promoting overall life satisfaction and success.

So let's delve into resilience.

Source:

Mayo Clinic Staff. "Positive thinking: Stop negative self-talk to reduce stress." Mayoclinic.org. November, 21, 2023. https://mayocl.in/3w6MBiC

RESILIENCE

"Life plays with you, doesn't it? And if you can manage it, you have to battle it. It's a jungle out there."

— Barbara Dreyfuss, *Lives Well Lived* film star, age 92

What is resilience? The fourth key element in a life well lived has to be resilience. All the people I interviewed had it, and I certainly believe it to be a critical component in being successful in your life—however you define success. We are all cognizant of the fact that life isn't a Hollywood movie. It is rare to be rich and famous. It is rare to become globally recognized or to be a national champion in some endeavor. Yet, irrespective of our financial or celebrity status (or lack thereof), all of us can, will, and do impact the lives of those around us.

Equally, all of us encounter challenges and obstacles on the way to our goals. Many times, we overcome them; sometimes we don't. Being able to face those issues, challenges, and obstacles—and still flourish and prosper in life—is the very definition of resilience. Losing a partner. Saying goodbye to a loved one on a train station in an occupied country. Having a business enterprise go bankrupt. There were so many stunning examples of resilience in those I interviewed that I came to see this as an integral component of living a life well lived.

Perhaps one of the most poignant for me was when film star, Evy Justesen, talked about Viktor Frankl's book, *Man's Search for Meaning,* being a strong factor in her life. In the book, he writes about his time as a Holocaust survivor, and that he could not predict who would make it out alive based on their physical strength; rather, it was from their attitude. As he says in the book, "Everything can be taken from a man but one thing: the last of the human freedoms—to choose one's attitude in any given set of circumstances, to choose one's own way." He was living in an extreme time, but it is applicable for any situation.

Many times in our lives we cannot change the things that are happening around us, but what we can change is our attitude about how we deal with those events, even under dire circumstances. I thought about this often during the pandemic, when the world was collectively going through something very traumatic. The great thing about resilience is that anyone of any age can demonstrate it.

"It's not how many times you get knocked down that count, but how many times you get up."

(This quote has been reworked and attributed to many, but is thought to have originally come from Confucius.)

Many of the film stars were amazingly resilient, especially through World War II. I will focus briefly on two of the stories. As a child growing up in Latvia, Emmy Cleaves and her mother were forced to flee when the Russians invaded their small village. After escaping a forced labor camp, Emmy (age 15) and her mother ran to the train station, bombs falling around them. They made it to the station; her mother jumped on the train, but while Emmy was handing her their bags, the doors closed, separating them. The train departed, leaving Emmy alone on the platform. It would be another twelve years before mother and daughter would learn if the other had survived. Her message of resilience, "Never become a victim, because there is always hope."

Susy Eto Bauman's story is yet another moving example of enduring strength and resilience. Born in the United States and having never visited Japan, she was interned during World War II, along with approximately 120,000 other Japanese Americans due to her Japanese heritage. Despite this, her husband chose to join the army (442nd Infantry Regiment) to demonstrate his loyalty to the country. Susy, fearing for his safety, advised against it, but he was determined to prove his allegiance.

Tragically, her fears were realized when her husband was killed in action. This devastating loss sent Susy into a deep depression, grappling with the daunting task of single parenthood. During this period, she struggled with the will to continue living, weighed down by sorrow. Yet, it was the support and encouragement from her friends, urging her to persevere for her children's sake, that helped her emerge from her despair. Gradually, she discovered inner strength and her and her reflective wisdom from that period became, "Life is not easy; there are lots of obstacles. You have to be strong enough and have a positive way of thinking, so that you can overcome anything that comes your way."

I've realized, after reflecting on the idea of resilience (informed by discussions with the people in my documentary) that resilience isn't something you are born with, an innate trait. Rather, it is something you earn and learn through life's experiences. Newborns start life reliant on their parents' support. As they grow, engaging in play and exploration, they develop physical strength and coordination. Inevitably, they experience falls and minor injuries like scraped knees, causing temporary discomfort. Yet, they bounce back, demonstrating the body's capacity to heal and recover.

As we navigate through life, we might accumulate scars, both literally and metaphorically. Looking at my own hands and knees, I see evidence of life's trials. Resilience is akin to a muscle or our skin; it strengthens through overcoming challenges. Though these experiences might leave us bruised or scarred, they also make us more robust. This was a common thread in the stories of those with whom I spoke.

Their resilience came from overcoming adversity. Each challenge they surmounted boosted their confidence and resilience. A positive mindset and intentional choices were crucial, yet the standout quality that was their key trait was perseverance. They didn't surrender; instead, they continually got back up, metaphorically remounting the horse after each fall. Don't be afraid to take on that challenge—even if it is a little daunting. That challenge may be exactly what you need to toughen up that resilience muscle a little more.

Then, the next time you are challenged in a similar way, it might just seem a little easier. No one goes from budding athlete to Olympian in one step or in an instant. Unfortunately, in the modern world, we are sold the idea of the magic silver bullet: the one pill that cures our ills or helps us 'get rich quick.' I believe we should all turn our backs on this instant, quick-fix philosophy of the modern world. Maybe this saying is somewhat extreme—but you may have heard it:

"That which does not kill us makes us stronger."

— Friedrich Nietzsche

It seems clear to me that all the people I interviewed had a rich and well-lived life because they 'lived it.' They met challenges; they gave their time and love to others; they found a purpose, and they considered the positive outlook. It was exactly this combination of doing, of work, of living—that added up to a life well lived. Trying to do things easy—to win instantly—might seem fun, but in the end, you might well be cheating yourself out of the experiences and wisdom along the way.

I am sure all of us know of a famous or less famous example of this. Perhaps it is a single mother you know who took on the raising of her kids after a divorce or the loss of a husband. Maybe it is someone who survived an extreme weather event or who volunteered every summer fighting fires or flood, all the time risking their lives. Do they not seem just a little more alive than others who had an easy life? Building resilience doesn't necessarily mean such a huge, earth-shattering event. In fact, for many of us, it may be much more mundane. Little, everyday challenges build up over a life where our ability grows, step by step, along the way.

The stories of those who have navigated life's twists and turns with courage and optimism remind us that true strength lies in our capacity to endure and grow. As we continue our own journeys, let us embrace each obstacle not as a setback, but as an opportunity to strengthen our resilience, deepen our wisdom, and enrich our lives. In doing so, we not only enhance our own life's narrative but also inspire those around us to find the beauty and strength in their own challenges.

How can you become more resilient? Building resilience, the ability to adapt well in the face of adversity, trauma, tragedy, threats, or significant sources of stress, is a crucial skill for navigating life's challenges. Here are key steps to help you become more resilient:

- **Develop strong relationships.** Cultivate supportive relationships and have caring and supportive people around.
- Foster wellness. Take care of your body through regular exercise, balanced nutrition, sufficient sleep, and mindfulness practices like meditation or yoga. Mindfulness practices can help you stay grounded and focused on the present moment.
- **Cultivate a positive outlook.** I believe optimism and resilience go hand in hand. Optimism enables you to expect that good things will happen. Look for silver linings, even in tough situations.
- **Embrace change and be proactive.** The only constant is change. Be open to staying flexible and adaptable. When things are changing, be proactive, make a plan, and take action.
- **Learn from experiences.** Tough times are often the periods in which we learn the most about ourselves. Reflect on past experiences, both positive and negative. Learning from past challenges can increase your confidence in being more resilient. Recognizing when you cannot handle a situation on your own and seeking help is a sign of strength, not weakness. Setting realistic and achievable goals gives you a sense of purpose and direction. Break these goals down into manageable steps.
- **Keep things in perspective.** Try to view stressful situations in a broader context. Avoid blowing events out of proportion and maintain a long-term perspective.

Developing resilience is a personal journey, and what works for one person, might not work for another. It's about finding what strategies resonate with you and incorporating them into your life.

WORDS OF WISDOM FROM OUR FILM STARS

I consider myself incredibly fortunate to have had the privilege of capturing the stories of many remarkable individuals in the *Lives Well Lived* documentary. These stories range from those of Holocaust survivors to music teachers who have nurtured world-class musicians, from sculptors to family cooks, and from artists to dreamers. They come from diverse walks of life, representing a colorful spectrum of experiences. You can find a curated selection of film star biographies that offer deeper insights into their lives and perspectives on our website:

www.lives-well-lived.com/bios

Here, I offer you my favorite words of wisdom from these remarkable individuals.

My firm belief is that everyone has a story to tell if we just take the time to listen.

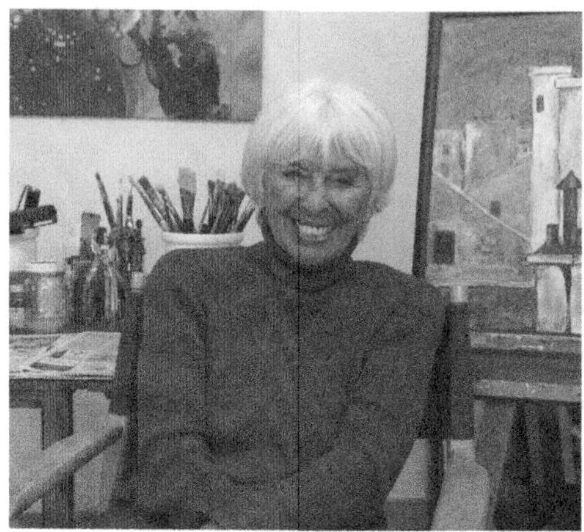

"What is really important in life is taking chances, risking, facing new situations, learning new skills and not getting in a rut. The attitude you have about life is really the only thing you have control over, and that is what determines how you are going to live your life."

—Evy Justesen, Age 81

"Happiness is a state of mind. You can be happy with what you have, or miserable with what you don't have. You decide."

—Lou Tedone, Age 92

Lou's philosophy:
"Help a lot of people.
Do the best you can."

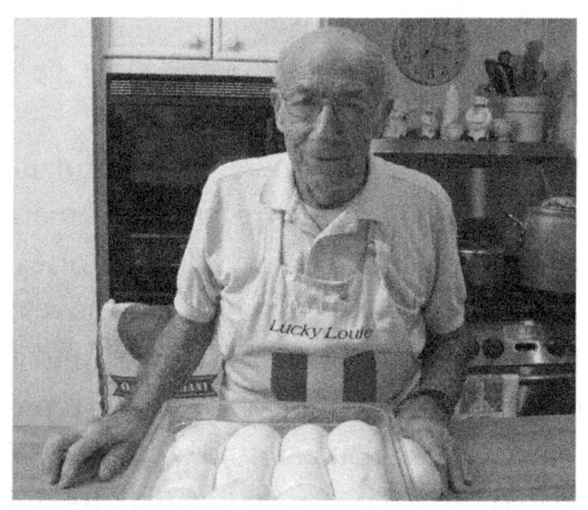

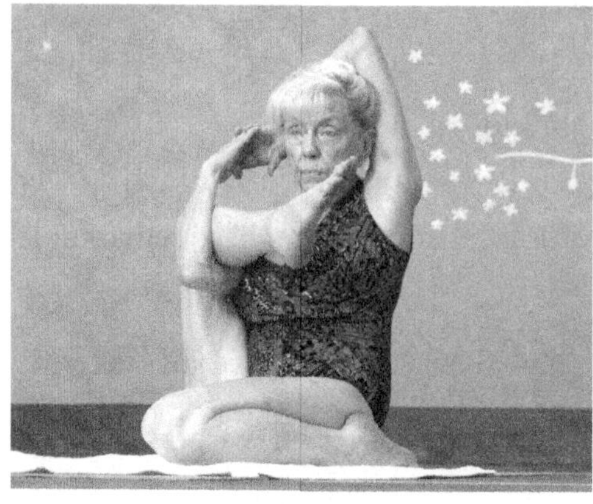

"The secret for a happy life is to really enjoy what you have and what you are doing, not to continuously be dissatisfied. Don't yearn for things; they don't make you happy."

—Emmy Cleaves, Age 86

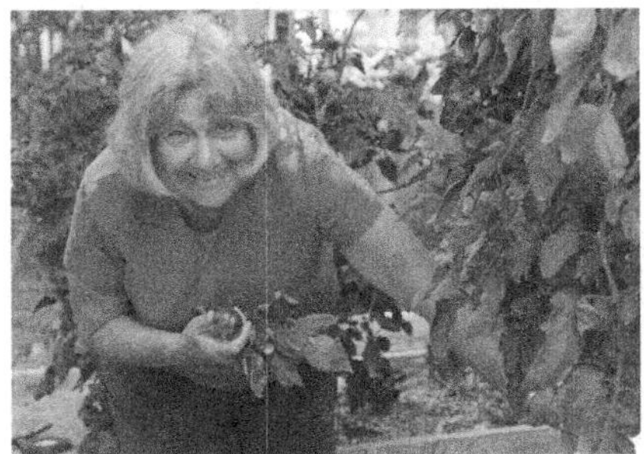

"It's really important that you make the most out of every day; you never know what tomorrow will bring. You can't get out of life if you don't put anything into life. It's like anything else. There's no free ride."

—Marion Woflf, Age 84

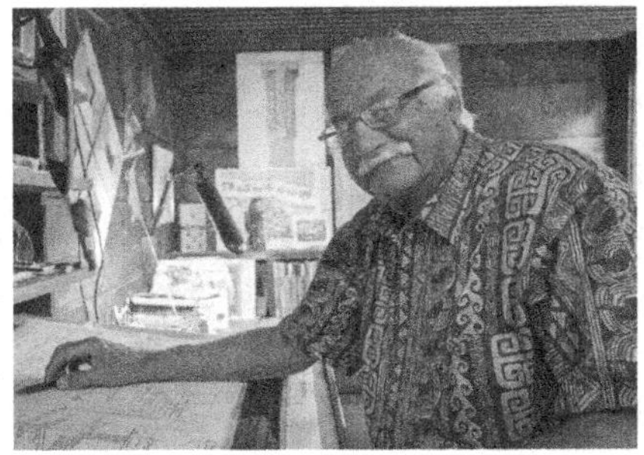

"I realize that I've got far less life ahead of me than behind me, but I'm not at the stage where I'm particularly concerned with that. I'm much more concerned with trying to get the most out of life as it is for me today."

—Paul Wolff, Age 84

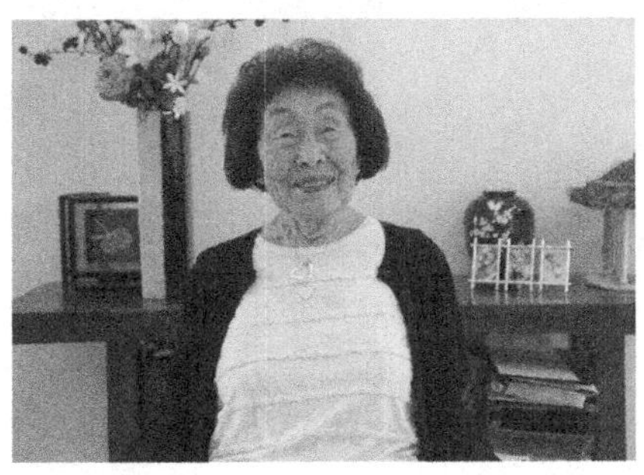

"A lot of my friends say, 'Oh, I'm getting too old, I can't do this. I can't do that.' But I say, 'phooey with that.' If I want to do something, I do it. If you say, 'I can't do it,' then you won't be able to do it. Just go out and do it."

—Susy Eto Bauman, Age 95

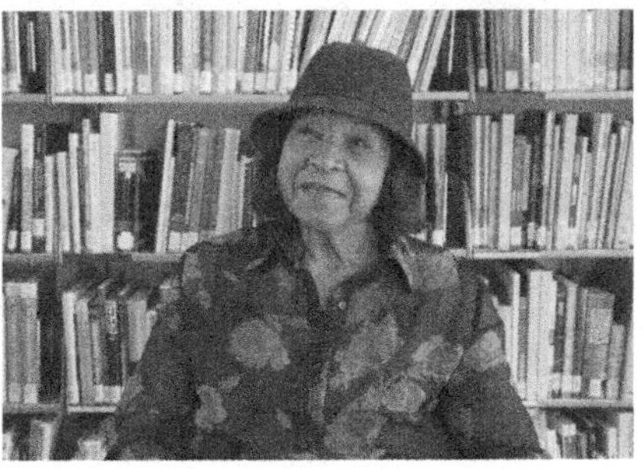

"Even I though I'm 80, I still want to finish my Ph.D. I have six more units at USC. No matter what age you are, learning never stops. You still keep learning."

—Rose Albano Ballestero, Age 80

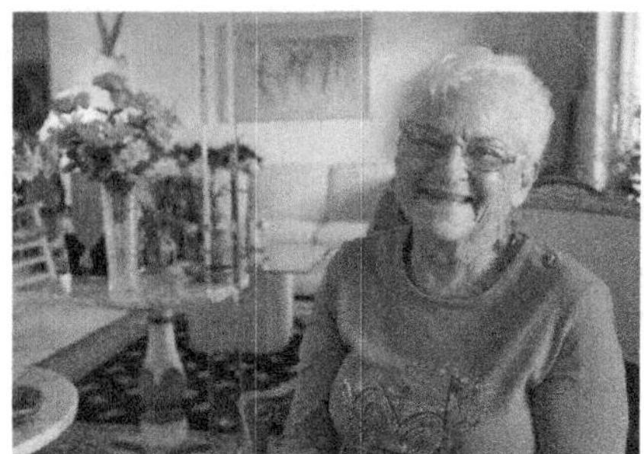

"Live one day at a time. Tomorrow comes soon enough."

—Irene Devin, age 90

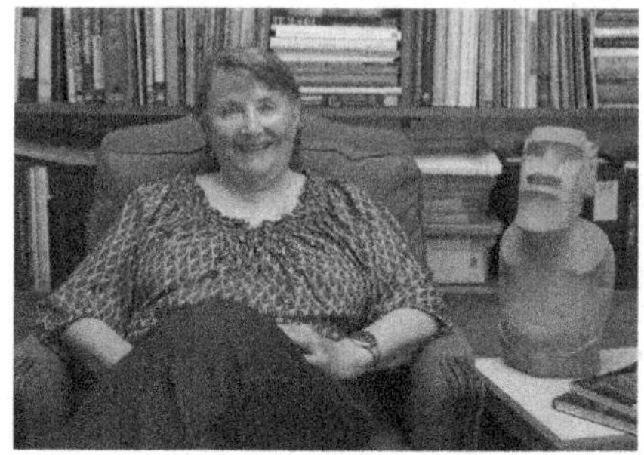

"I've always felt you need to sit loosely in the saddle of life as you go down that long trail."

—Georgia Lee, age 87

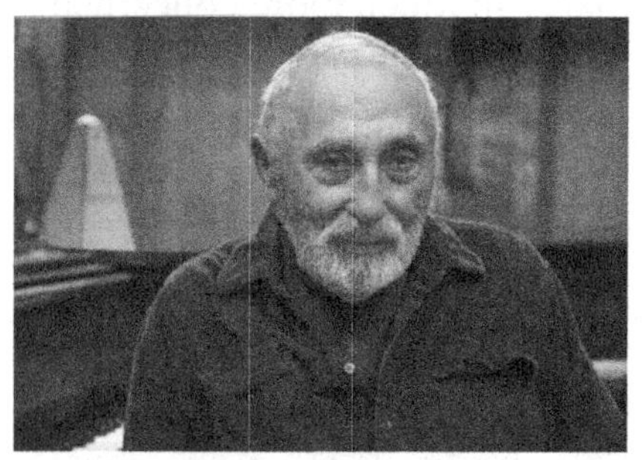

"I respect yesterday, what is history. Today, I look at things realistically. And tomorrow I dream."

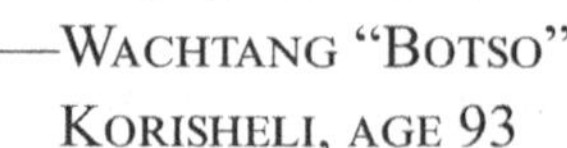

—Wachtang "Botso" Korisheli, age 93

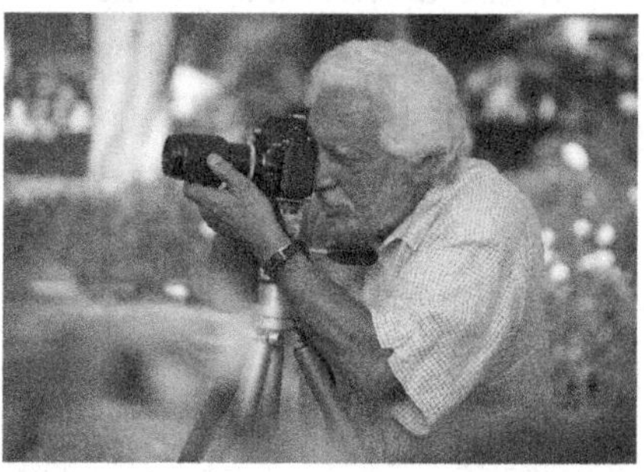

"An Indian chief once said, 'You will be remembered by the tracks you leave behind,' and I'm trying to leave good tracks."

—Santi Visalli, age 81

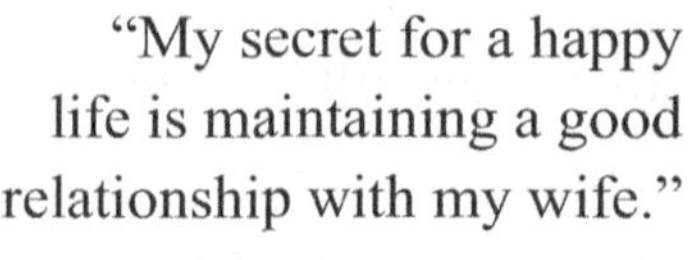

"My secret for a happy life is maintaining a good relationship with my wife."

—Bob Cleaves, age 84

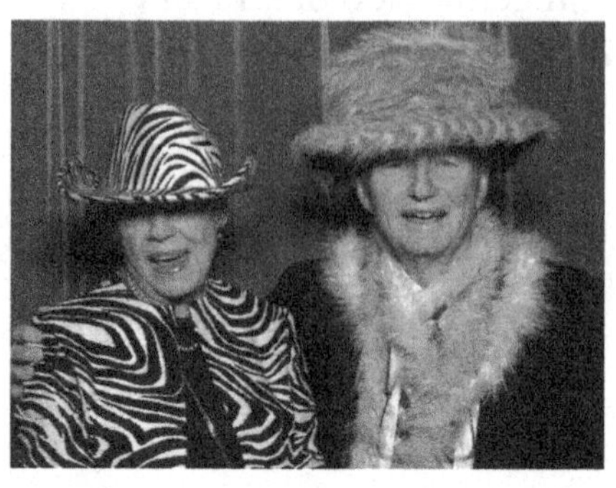

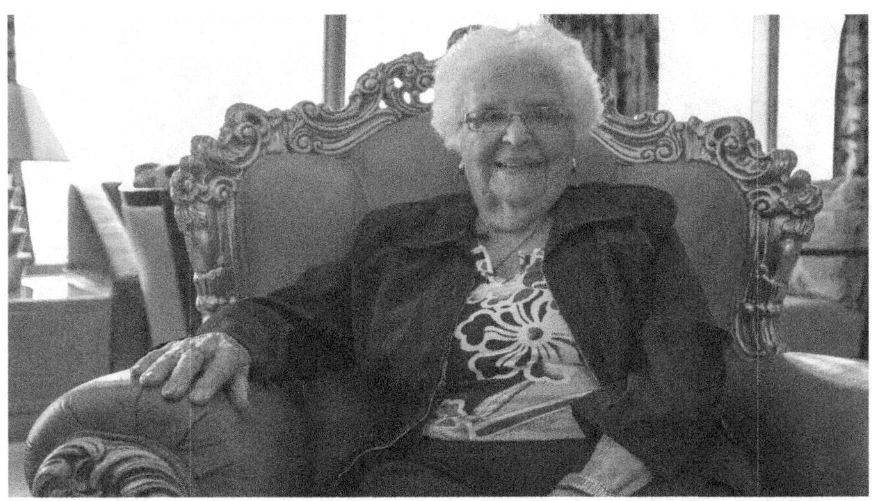

"In my lifetime, I don't think I ever made an enemy because I always tried to help, I always gave what I could, and I made friends very easily. I feel being kind and being nice to people, no matter where you are, no matter what situation, it always comes back to you. It's a wonderful way to be in life. That's my philosophy of life."

—Evelyn Ricciuti, Age 103

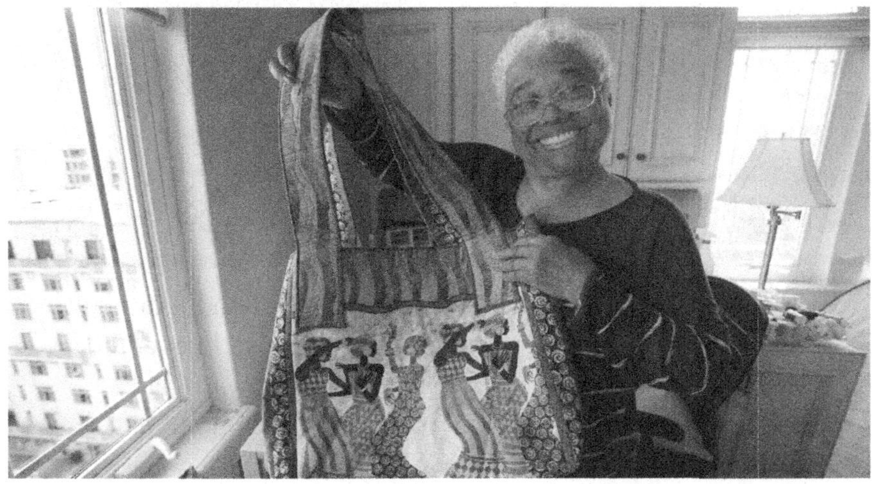

"Life goes by so quickly, and most young people are in such a hurry to get to the next part of their life (or wherever they're going), that they don't really take time to just enjoy what's happening right now." —Blanche Brown, Age 78

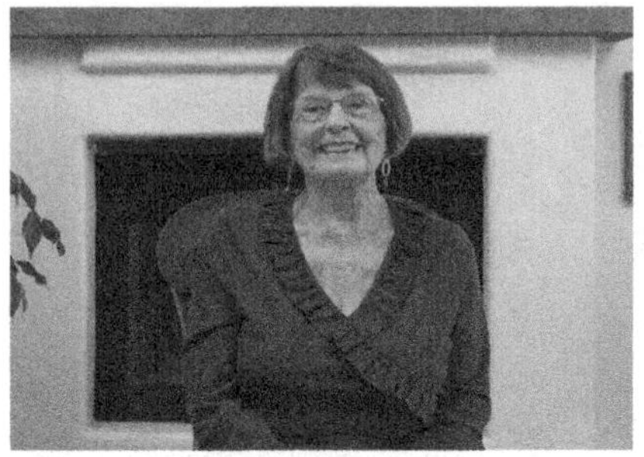

"At 81, I think I'm probably more comfortable in my own skin. You worry so much when you're younger about what other people think, needless worry. When you're 81, you can be a little outrageous now and then and get away with it. You should have fun!"

—Dottie Thompson, age 81

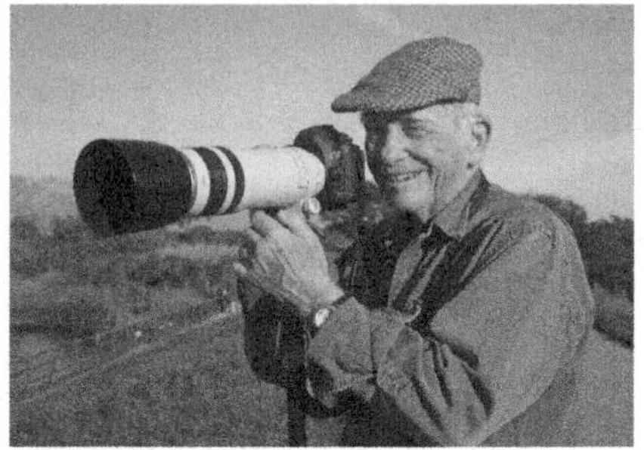

"You wonder, 'how much longer can I travel' or 'how much longer can I exercise like I like to exercise?' It's called *futurizing*, and it's stupid. Don't worry what's down the road, live in the moment."

—Jesse Alexander, age 85

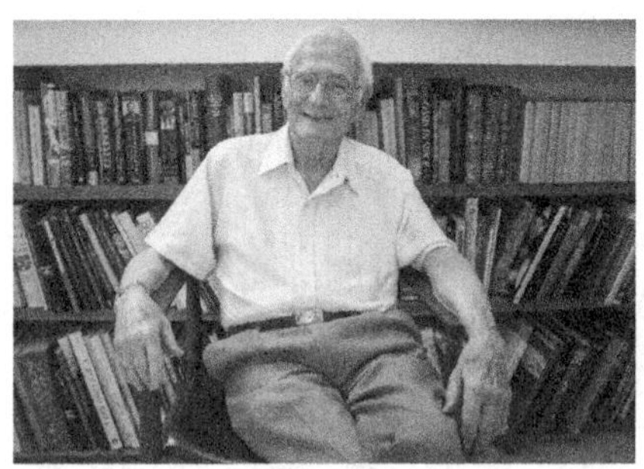

"I wish younger people would understand that you need to be more tolerant. Different people have different points of view about the world. You can't just impose your views on everyone else."

—Bob Sinsheimer, age 90

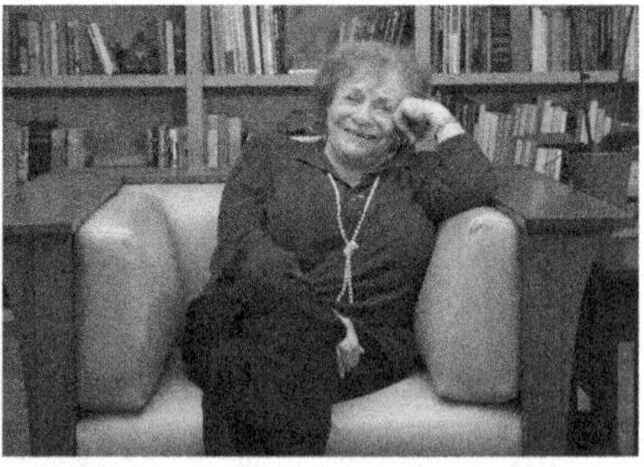

"I know that I find it difficult to live alone, so I never did live alone. I always had a partner and sought to have a partner, and was quite successful with it, I must say."

—Barbara Dreyfuss, age 91

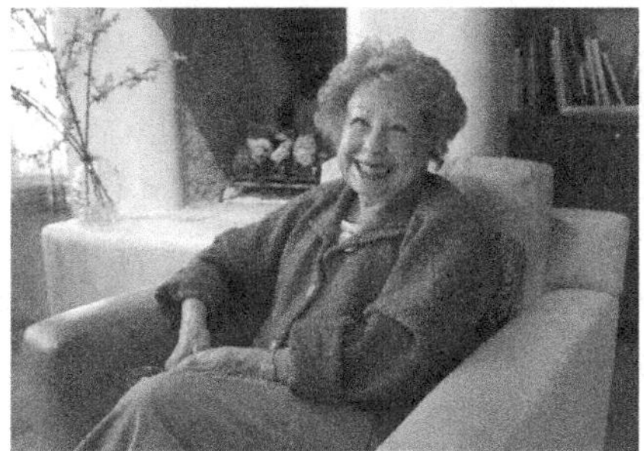

"One thing that I have learned is how important it is to let go of anger. I see people that are holding on to grudges for years and years, and it just pollutes your life. And I think that living in the moment, enjoying each day, is very important."

—BRENDA EDELSON, AGE 75

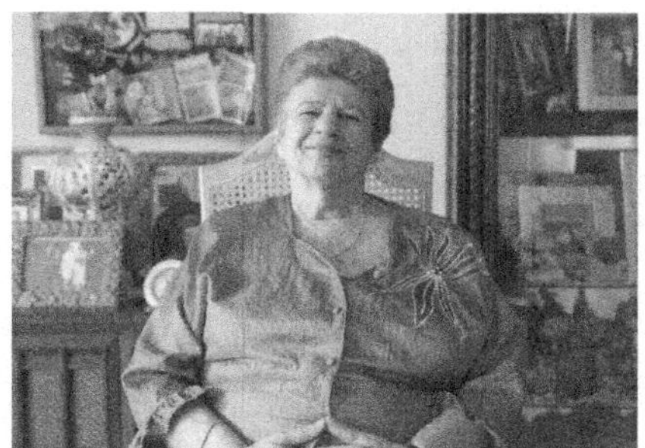

"I've been given all these days and years, which I've embraced because I see life as incredibly precious. I hardly ever said 'no' to anything, I just made sure that every day was filled with joy, purpose, and meaning."

—BARBARA GESINO, AGE 75

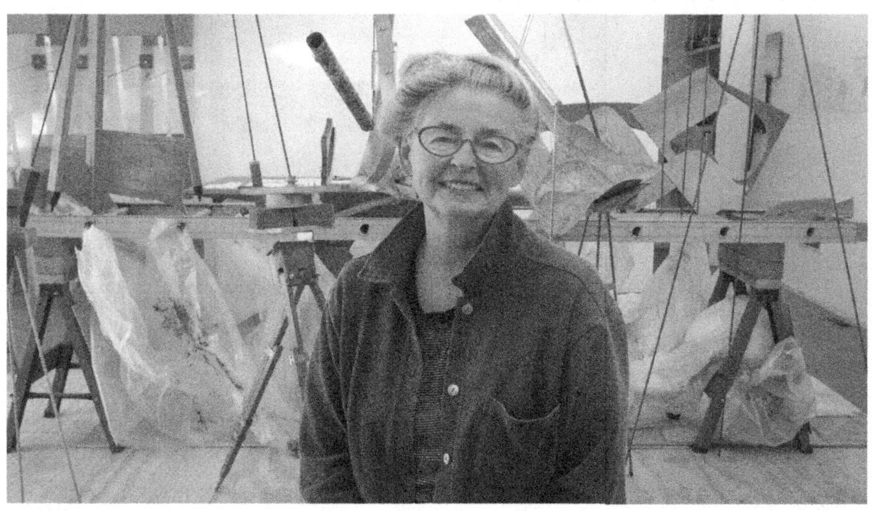

"When I was younger, I wish I had known that I could have been more courageous."

—JOAN TANNER, AGE 78

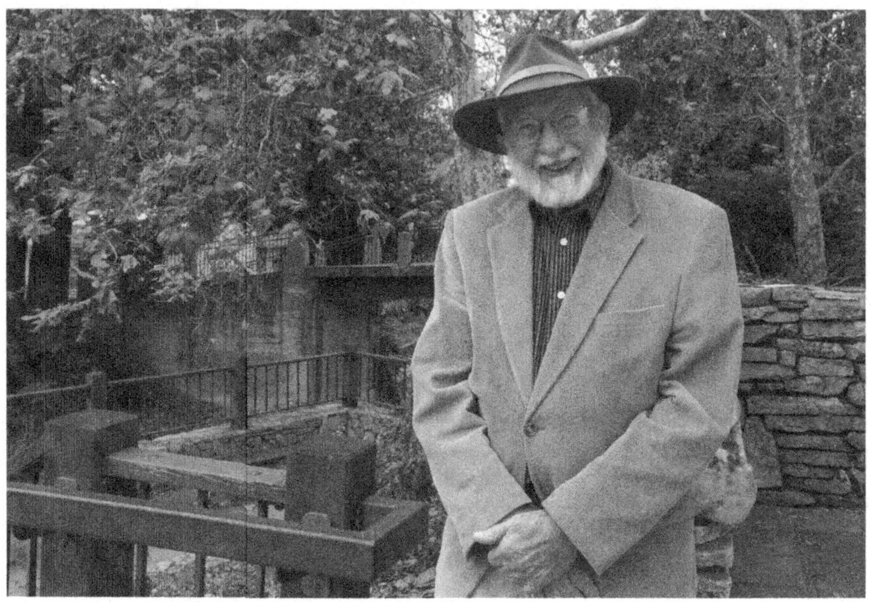

"A life well lived? Perhaps knowing when to say 'no' to certain opportunities and when to say 'yes' to certain ones that might sound a little iffy."

—Ken Schwartz, age 90

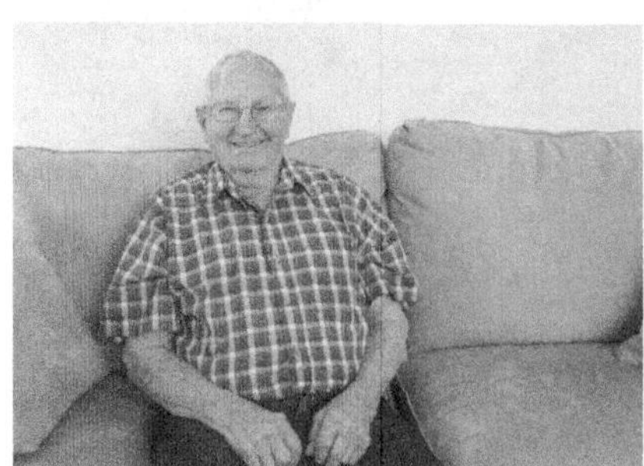

"I think the key to a person living a long time is being happy and not worrying so much about things, because worrying can kill anybody."

—Eugene Pozzebon, age 89

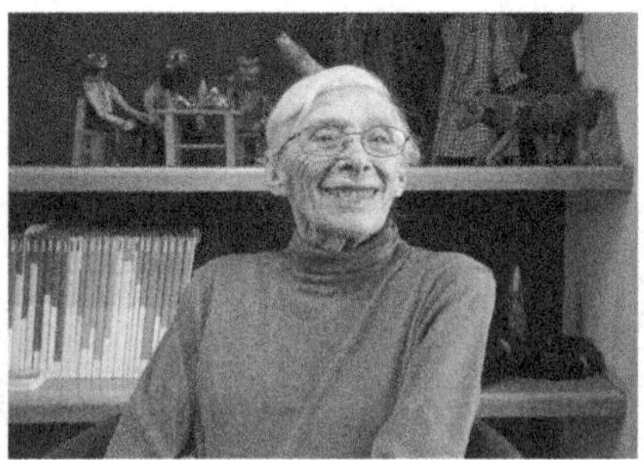

"My definition of a life well lived? Do something useful, have a social conscience, and try to work for a better world in whatever way you can."

—Terry Hertz, Age 95

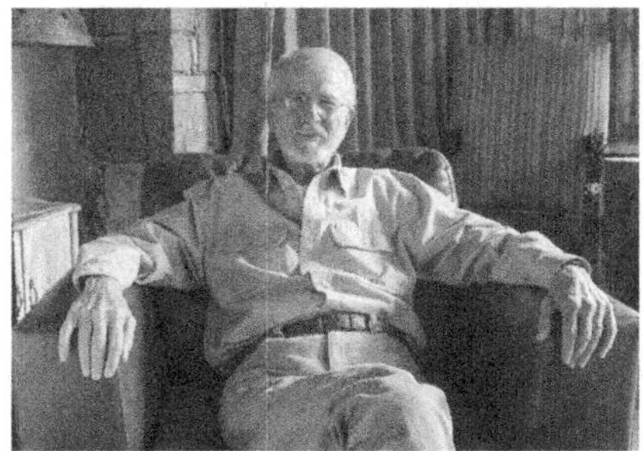

"One of my favorite songs is 'Enjoy Yourself, It's Later Than You Think.' The years go by really quickly, so—enjoy it while you're 'still in the pink.' as they say in the song."

—Joe Stevens, age 78

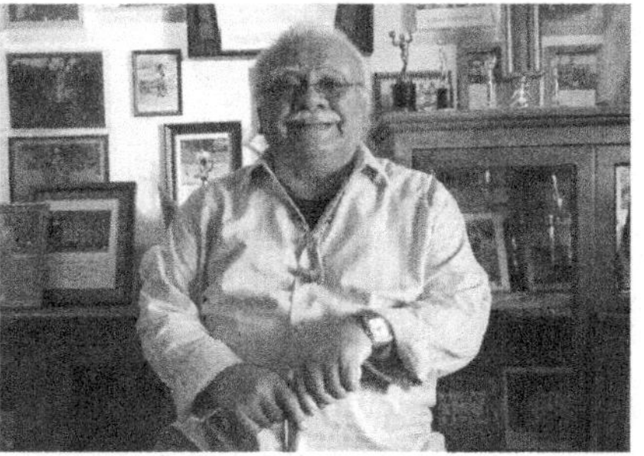

"I think people need to learn to be patient and understanding. I think they should the appreciate life."

—Joe Talaugon, age 83

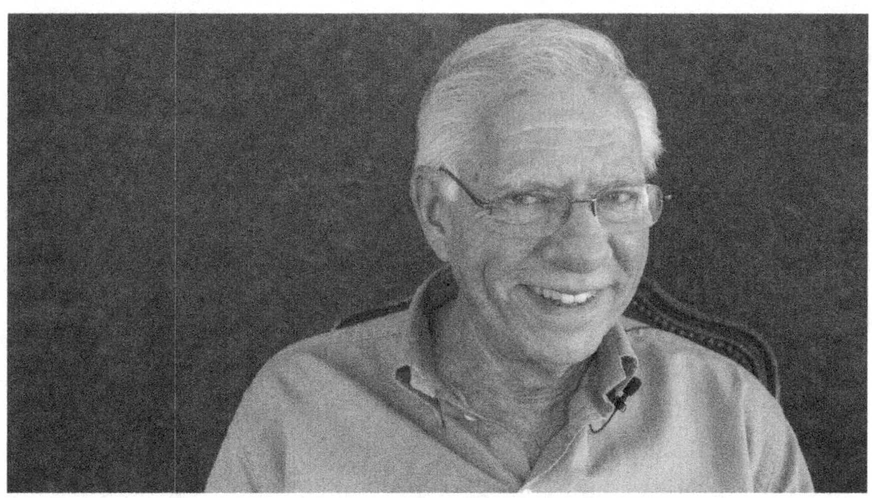

"A life well lived, for me, means having lived life to the fullest. I think I was always moving ahead, never stagnating, always trying to look for something different. And trying to achieve a goal that sometimes was not achievable. I've often said that I thank God for putting obstacles in my way because I think I learn from overcoming every obstacle."

—Herbert Bergman, age 75

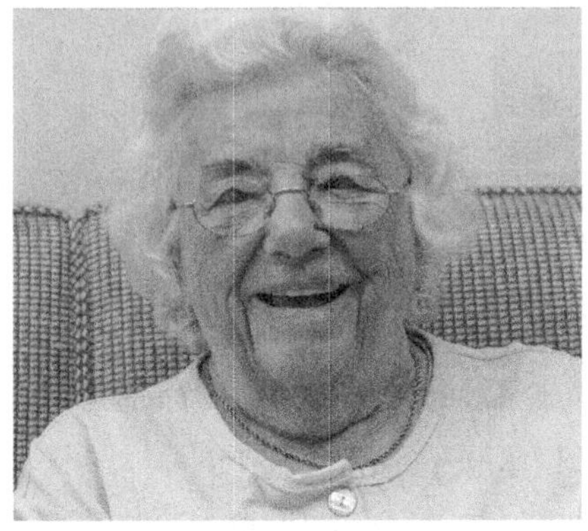

"Don't sweat the little things. Do the best you can."

—Doris Achterkirchen, Age 97

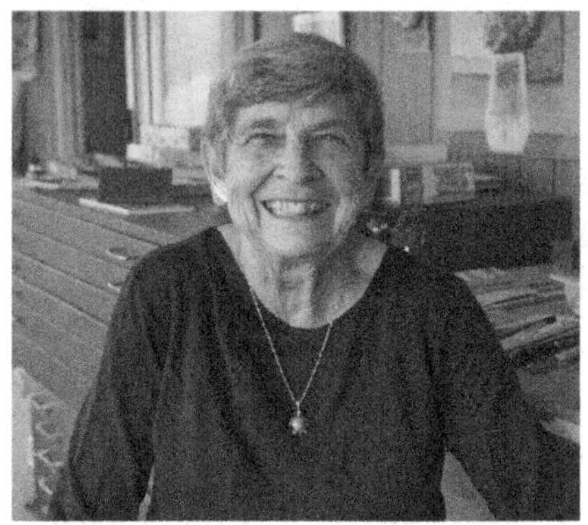

"I feel a life well lived is probably just being endlessly engaged in whatever your passion is."

—Rachael Winn Yon, Age 78

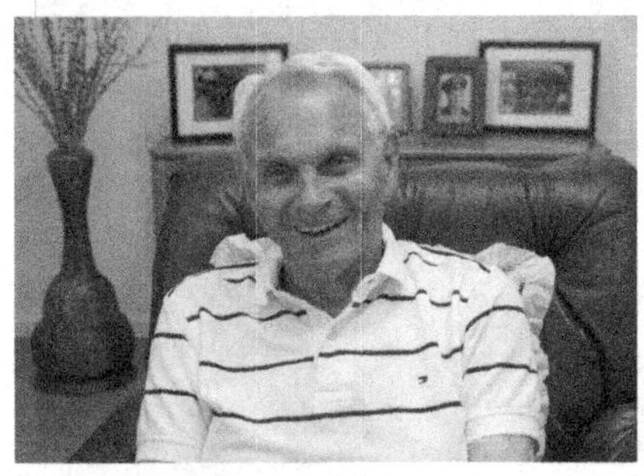

"I don't think people should worry about getting old because they're going to get old. You can't stop birthdays, and you're going to keep getting older every year. But you don't have to be old, mentally."

—Lou Goodman, Age 90

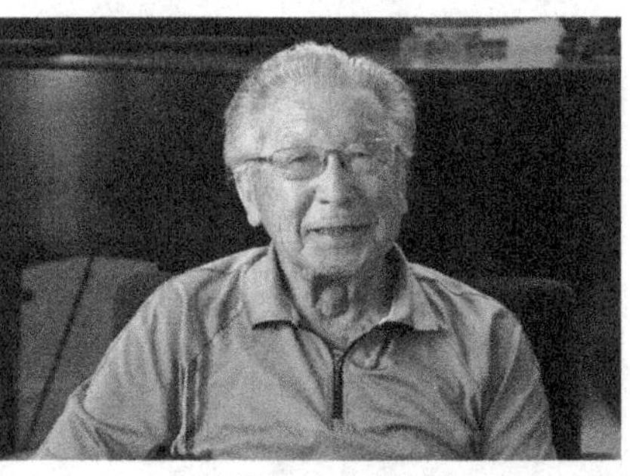

"I wished, when I was younger, I would not have been as rowdy and caused my mother a lot of headaches and what not. I outgrew that because, as you grow older, you become more tolerant and more compassionate."

—Satoshi Hane, Age 91

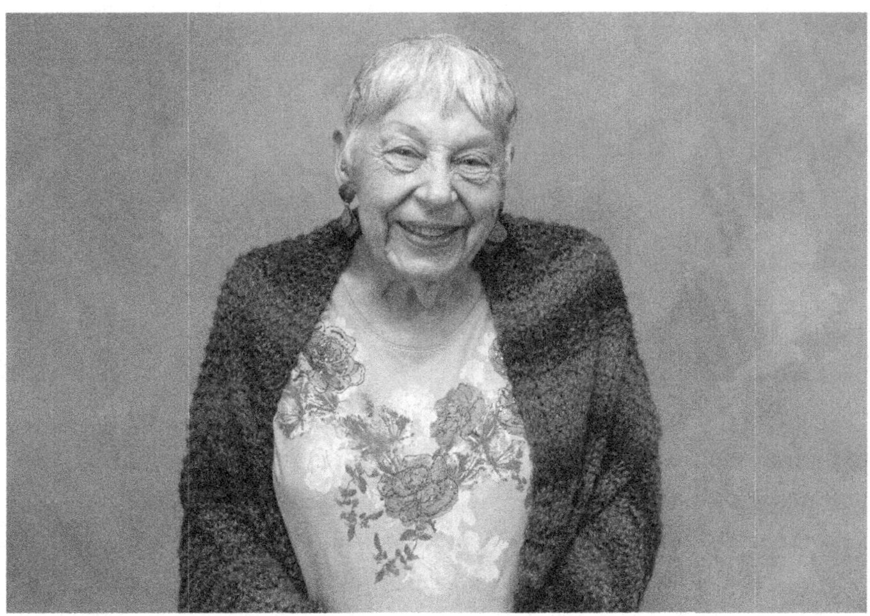

"The best advice that I ever received came from my Sunday school teacher, and she said, 'There's so much good in the worst of us, and so much bad in the best of us, it hardly behooves any of us to talk about the rest of us.' And I think that I've lived my life with that realization, and I've always looked for the good in people."

—Barbara J. Williams, age 85

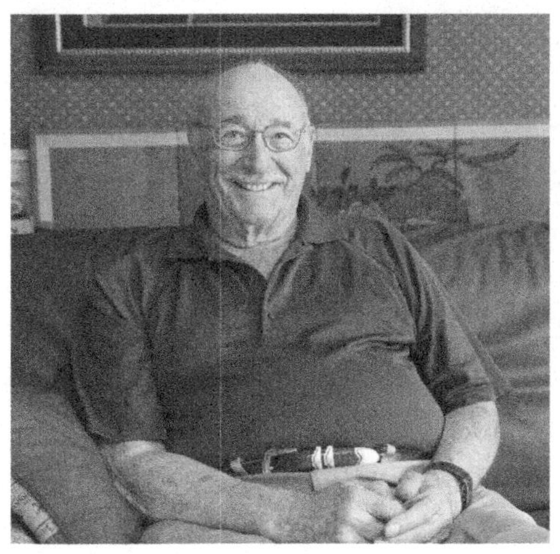

"I think the biggest thing people should *not* worry about is failure. I think failure is a great teacher."

—William Abel, age 85

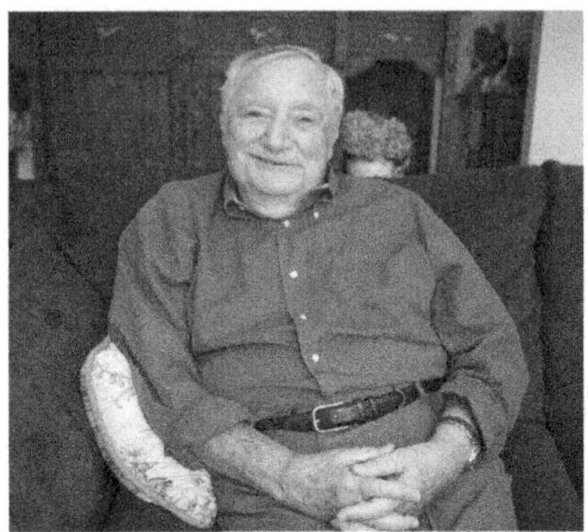

"Luck has the aroma of perspiration. You don't get lucky without working very hard for things."

—JULES HOCK, AGE 79

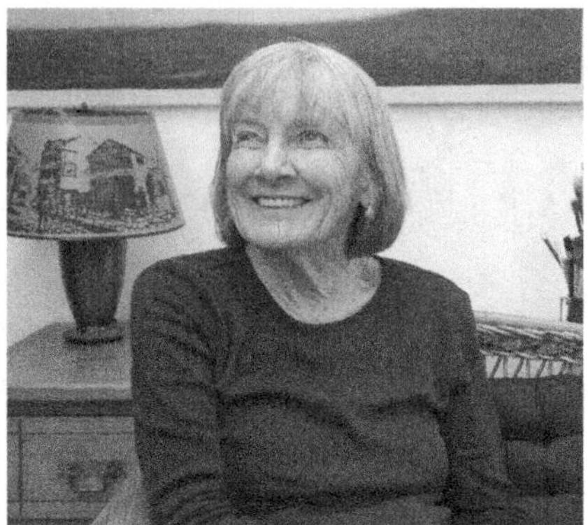

"I think what keeps me going is my own internal curiosity. People will say to me, you're so curious."

—LINNAEA PHILLIPS, AGE 81

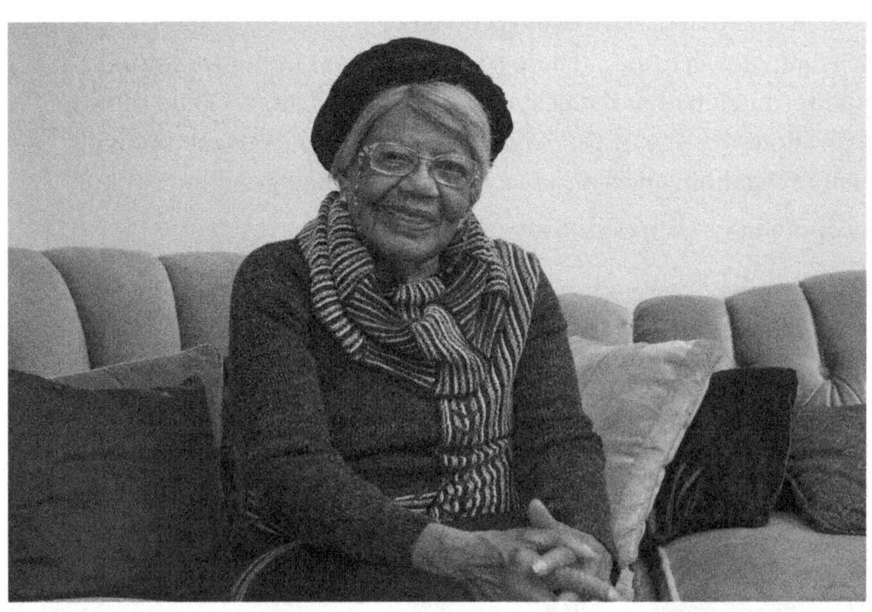

"I have always been surrounded by lots of friends. I love to meet new people. And I phrase it, 'I don't meet strangers.'"

—JESSIE STONE, AGE 84

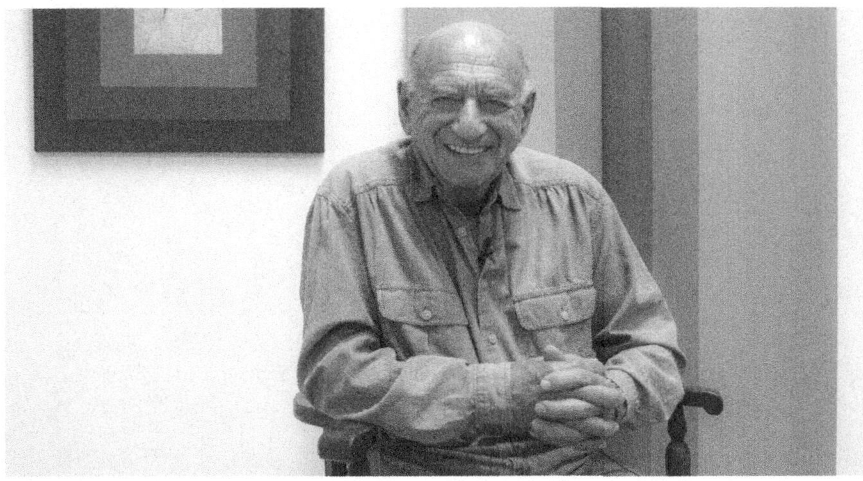

"Work a little less. Spend a little less. Enjoy life a little more."

—Dr. Edward Okun, age 82

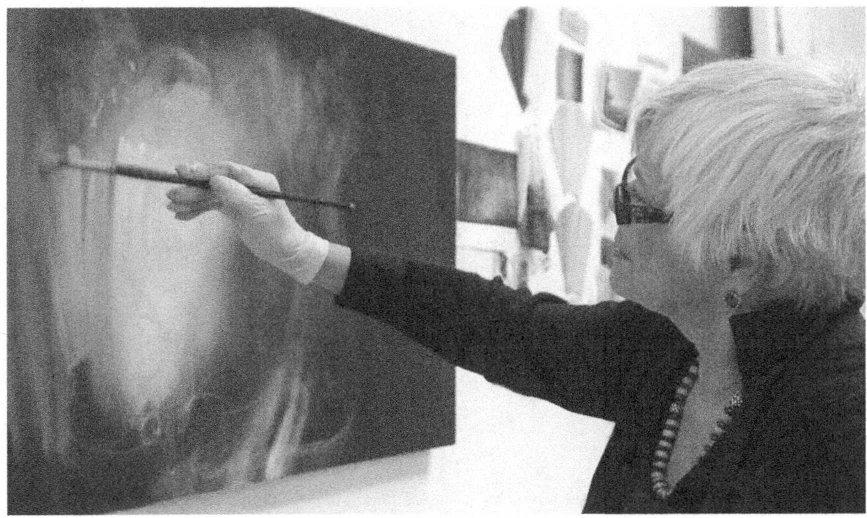

"Probably the most important thing in a relationship is absolute honesty and absolute respect of the other. What I've learned is to never try to change anyone, not one iota. The only person who can adjust is yourself. Leave the other person totally alone, that's very important to know. I wish I had known that when I was very young. You try to help or try to change; none of that works. We are each the imperfect beauty that we are."

—Ciel Bergman, Age 76

CAPTURING THE STORIES OF OLDER ADULTS IN YOUR LIFE

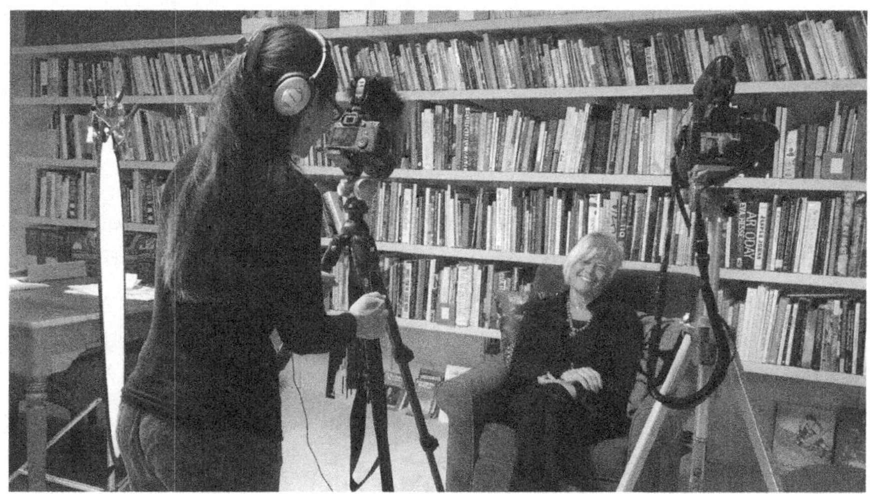

Interviewing an older adult in your life is an endeavor filled with profound moments and cherished connections. One of the questions I asked all the participants of the film was, "Do you have any regrets?" The most common response was their regret of not having asked more questions to those who had passed away. It's a common illusion to think we have endless time, only to find out we don't. I've found that interviewing someone close to you, be it a family member, a friend, or a mentor, is a profoundly touching experience. It might seem intimidating at first (I know it was for me), but believe me, you can do it!

I like to say that I have forty new grandparents as a result of working on the film. Most of the interviewees have become close friends since our experience filming together. In many cases, I learned more about them than about family members. Why? Because I took the time to ask questions and to be an active listener. And isn't that the way? You talk with someone, learn more about them, and you build a bond with them while they share their lives and their wisdom? If you don't take the time, you don't ever get to know them, and in my view, that is an opportunity missed.

Tips for interviews…

Remember, you don't have to create a video or film. You can interview people taking notes with pen and paper, record an audio interview or simply sit and listen.

1. Start with a framework. The most difficult part of an interview is having a framework, a starting point for the conversation. I will never forget bringing a student assistant, James, with me to interview Lucky Louie. Now, if you knew Lou, he was just an amazing guy and quite the storyteller. After we left the interview, James said to me, "Wow, I did not know older people could talk so much."

I asked James, "Do you have an older adult in your life?" He said that he had a grandfather, but they were not close since they did not live near to each other, but they were going to see one another that weekend because of a family get-together. So, being his teacher, I gave him an assignment: take the questions that we had just asked Lucky Louie and ask them to his grandfather.

Well, he came back from that trip grinning from ear to ear. His grandfather was delighted that he took an interest and wanted to know more about him and his life. Both the grandson and grandfather wanted to have a closer relationship and to get to know each other better, but they did not know where to begin. Having the questions in hand gave them both the space to get to know each other better and to begin to develop a relationship.

Starter questions: Are you wondering where to begin? Here are a few questions to get the conversation start:

- *What is your definition of a life well lived?*
- *What do you attribute to living as long as you have?*
- *What do you wish younger people understood about life?*
- *What is your secret to a happy life?*
- *What do you think about your own mortality?*

2. Create a sense of ease. For my project, I had to learn how to video and record people from scratch. Sure, I'm a professional photographer, but film is a whole other level of complexity. My grandmother was a good sport about being in front of the camera and being my first subject. Most of us don't spend a lot of time with a camera in our face. And frankly, no one really likes it, or ever gets used to it. So, when I interview someone, especially someone I'm not familiar with, I always take time to make them feel at ease. A few days before the interview, I like to meet them, just for a casual chat, without any camera gear. This helps build a comfortable rapport. I've learned that if the person I'm interviewing isn't relaxed, it really shows in the video. **Creating that personal connection is key even before the interview starts.** It is an artificial environment, and yet, you want it to look and sound as natural as possible—just a one-on-one conversation between friends in front of a camera and a microphone.

I approach every interview like an athlete preparing for a big game; warming up is essential. I don't dive straight into the questions. I start filming during the setup because often the most genuine moments happen when the person doesn't realize the camera is on. They're just themselves, which is what I'm looking for. Before an interview, I ask the person to send a bio and answer some questions in advance. This helps me understand them better and guides the direction of the interview. It's all about creating a comfortable, authentic conversation; these steps help me achieve that.

3. Set the expectations (but remain flexible). I always make it a point to explain to the interviewee what I'm looking for and why I'm interviewing them. This helps them give clearer, more focused answers. I **prepare thoroughly for each interview, researching the person even if I already know them,** but I remain flexible. Sometimes people will throw out a curveball, a piece of information that you didn't expect. Be willing to go with the flow. An unexpected answer can take the interview in a completely new and interesting direction, and I'm always ready to follow that lead.

During the interview, I make sure there's enough space for the person to breathe and think. This not only helps in editing but sometimes leads to them sharing something unexpectedly profound. I also avoid 'yes' or 'no' questions, as they often end the conversation abruptly. Instead, **I frame questions to encourage a more expansive response.** I listen carefully for that perfect soundbite, the essence of what I'm trying to capture. If I don't get it at first, I'll gently guide the conversation until I do. Sometimes, I might even pretend there was a glitch with my audio gear to get them to repeat a particularly good point.

4. Be mindful of sound quality. On the more technical side, if you are going to create a video, then the most important part of video is *sound*! While visuals are undoubtedly crucial, audio quality often takes precedence. As a visual person, this was an interesting lesson to learn. Think about your own experience. How many times have you watched a video on the internet, where the image quality is less than perfect? You will stick with it if you can hear the audio. On the flip side, if you have excellent image quality and bad audio, no one will watch the story you have created. People will forgive bad image quality, but they will not forgive bad sound.

For the best sound, try to use an external microphone for your subject. For most interviews, using a lavalier mic is an easy way to significantly enhance audio quality. These mics are compact and unobtrusive, often going unnoticed by the person wearing them. A great advantage is their compatibility with smartphones, including iPhones, allowing for a high-quality audio recording without the need for expensive equipment. Such a setup is not only cost-effective but also elevates the sound quality beyond what standard camera or smartphone microphones offer. If you are using your smartphone for recording, remember to switch it to airplane mode. This simple step prevents interruptions, like incoming calls, ensuring your recording session remains undisturbed.

5. Choose your shooting location carefully. When choosing your location, listen to the noise that's in the room. Right now, close your eyes and take a moment to listen to the sound in your room. Every room has a certain subtle, often unnoticed background noise, which can include the hum of a refrigerator, the buzz of a light bulb, the whir of a computer fan, or just the natural acoustics of the space. This is called 'room tone.' When you can, try to find a place with the least amount of distracting noise. If there is a lot of noise, consider relocating. A simple trick I've learned for refrigerator noise is to place my car keys in the refrigerator if I need to unplug it to reduce noise, ensuring I don't forget to plug it back in later. (Or else I can't drive home!)

In more advanced situations, filmmakers will record room tone. The standard practice is to **capture about thirty seconds to one minute of ambient sound in the location, with all equipment set up as**

it would be during the actual recording. This is typically done in the quietest state of the room, with no active dialogue or movement. Everyone on set is usually asked to remain silent and still during this process to ensure a clean recording of the room's natural sound. In post-production, this room tone is then layered into the audio track to ensure a consistent and natural sound environment throughout the video or film.

Selecting a meaningful location for your interview can add depth to the storytelling, especially if the setting holds significance or resonates with the subject's experiences. Visually, **when I walk into an environment where I am going to film an interview, I am looking at two things: what is the light like, and what will be the best background to highlight the personality of the person I am interviewing?** The setting should complement your subject, accentuating their personality or the topic being discussed. There are times when the background is just too busy. In these cases, I opt for a plain background that allows your subject to stand out, or a backdrop that tells a story. The choice of location can significantly impact the mood and message of your interview.

6. Add visual impact in framing your shots. I prefer a shallow depth of field to keep the focus on the person, and I'm very mindful of the framing, often using the 'rule of thirds.' This technique involves imagining two horizontal and two vertical lines dividing the frame into nine equal parts. I position the interviewee, particularly their eyes, at one of the intersections of these lines. This creates a more engaging and balanced shot, making the viewer feel naturally drawn to the person speaking. It's a simple, yet effective way to add visual depth and interest to the interview.

When filming, I use a tripod for stability. Even if you are filming with a phone, you can get a very inexpensive little tripod. Shaky footage can be distracting, especially during interviews.

7. Use natural lighting when possible (and other lighting tips). Lighting plays a pivotal role in shaping the visual aesthetics of your interview. I love using natural light from a window if possible. However, it's crucial to avoid positioning your subject directly in front of a window, which can result in dark silhouettes. Instead, experiment with angles and placement to achieve the best possible lighting conditions. Where are you in relation to the subject? Sometimes it is as easy as moving around the subject to find the best light; sometimes you might have to move your subject into the best light. The more important thing is to just be mindful of the light as you are setting up your shot. In situations where natural light isn't available or sufficient, consider using additional lighting sources. An inexpensive LED light can be a valuable tool, or a five-in-one reflector that can bounce light onto your subject, softening shadows and creating a flattering effect.

8. Add B-Roll to create depth to the story. B-roll footage adds depth to the story. What is 'B-roll footage?' It refers to supplementary or cutaway footage that enhances the main interview content. Whether it's animation, photographs, or historical footage, it makes the final video more engaging. The most boring interviews that I have seen are filled with 'talking heads.' Using historical B-roll footage in your interviews can be a powerful storytelling tool, particularly when you're discussing events or topics with a rich historical context. For instance, if your interviewee is discussing a particular event or period in history, incorporating relevant historical footage can transport the audience back in time, immersing them in the historical context. This visual reinforcement can help viewers connect emotionally with the narrative and create a more immersive experience. Whether it's footage from a wartime era, a civil rights movement, or a pivotal moment in history, these visuals can elicit empathy, nostalgia, or a sense of awe.

The point is…

Capturing these stories, these life events, and these philosophies is worth all the effort in the end. So, as you embark on your interviewing journey, remember that it's not just about the technical aspects, but about celebrating the unique stories and personalities of those you interview. These moments are more than just interviews; they are like keys that unlock the doors to cherished chapters in the lives of your loved ones. Through the art of interviewing, you'll discover a treasure trove of shared experiences and profound insights, creating lasting bonds and treasured memories that will continue to inspire, educate, and warm the hearts of generations to come. Happy interviewing, and may your storytelling endeavors be filled with love, laughter, and meaningful connections.

For more tips about on interviewing and for a list of questions, go to:

 lives-well-lived.com/takeaction

THE INGREDIENTS OF A LIFE WELL LIVED

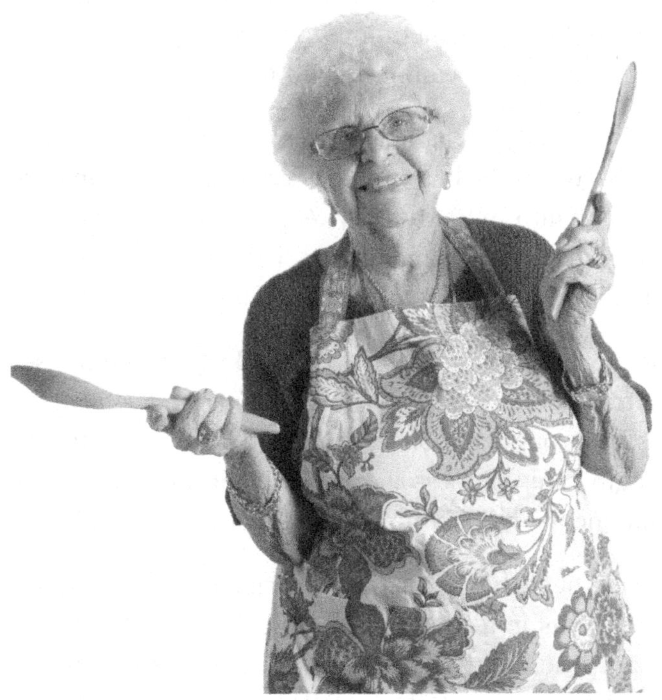

This project began in the kitchen with my grandmother sharing her life and wisdom while cooking up some delicious Italian recipes. I realize that in the art of living a fulfilling life, we can draw a striking parallel to the delicate process of cooking a memorable meal. Each element in this process corresponds to a vital component of a well-lived life.

Connection and support are much like the foundational stock or broth in a recipe. They provide the base, enriching and enhancing our life experiences, just as a well-prepared broth brings depth and sustenance to a dish. This foundational element nurtures and sustains us, offering strength and comfort from which we can grow and thrive.

Similarly, having a sense of purpose is akin to following a cherished family recipe. It gives us direction and clarity, ensuring that our actions and decisions come together in a harmonious blend. Like a recipe passed down through generations, a sense of purpose guides us toward creating something meaningful and fulfilling.

Positivity, in this culinary metaphor, serves as the seasoning. It is the art of adding just the right herbs or spices to a dish, transforming something ordinary into extraordinary. A positive outlook enhances our experiences, adding zest and flavor, helping us to savor each moment, and balancing out the more challenging aspects of life.

Finally, resilience is comparable to the cooking process itself. It represents the transformation of raw ingredients under heat, just as resilience transforms our experiences, both good and bad, into wisdom and inner strength. This process is essential, turning a collection of individual components into a complete and nourishing whole.

Together, these elements blend to create the rich tapestry of a life well lived. Like ingredients in a chef's dish, the balance and combination of connection, purpose, positivity, and resilience determine the quality of our lives. Each component is essential, contributing to the unique flavor and texture of the overall experience, much like the perfect meal, where every element comes together in a delightful harmony.

SECTION TWO

CONNECTING GENERATIONS

THE LIVES WELL LIVED INTERGENERATIONAL PROJECT: A FILMMAKER'S JOURNEY

Why focus on connecting generations? I was very lucky to have my grandmother in my life, yet realize many younger people don't have a positive connection with an older adult. The result is a rise in ageism, inherent in an age-segregated environment. I have observed this firsthand with my students at the university, many of whom have little to no interaction with an older adult outside of family. What I have learned is to combat any type of 'ism,' the first step is to cultivate a conversation and a connection—to truly see, hear, and value a person who is different from you.

The idea for an intergenerational project began with a desire to use the *Lives Well Lived* film to connect generations. Inevitably, when I held Q&A sessions after screenings, one common question that arose was, "How do we get young people to watch the film and get them more engaged with older adults?"

It took a bit of serendipity to get the *Lives Well Lived* Intergenerational Project off the ground. During a screening of my documentary at a local theater, a Psychology of Aging student from Cal Poly, San Luis Obispo, was inspired by the film. She went to her teacher, Professor Sara Bartlett, and said, "Wow, you need to see this film. It's exactly what you've been talking about in class." What made this even more remarkable was the discovery that Professor Bartlett and I both taught at the same university.

Bartlett recounted her experience watching the film: "I remember sitting in the theater with older adults on either side of me, completely engrossed in the movie. I was struck by how remarkable the individuals in the film were and the powerful message it conveyed about successful aging. As I sat there, I thought, *this film is something I need for my class.*" In that moment, Professor Bartlett, who had been teaching Psychology of Aging for several years, found the missing piece she had been searching for. Her goal was to reshape her students' perception of aging, dispel negative stereotypes, and inspire a more positive outlook.

Being faculty members at the same university paved the way to collaborate on a shared vision and led to the creation of the *Lives Well Lived* Intergenerational Project, a venture that began six years ago. The film was meant to challenge perceptions of aging, but its potential as a tool for intergenerational understanding was a new and exciting prospect. We envisioned an initiative that would bridge generations through shared stories and insights.

Initially, we worked with a local for-profit retirement community, the Villages of San Luis Obispo, where the film served as a catalyst for bringing students and older adults together. The film's portrayal of older adults in a positive light intrigued the students, sparking their curiosity about their older counterparts. Simultaneously, older adults who watched the film became enthusiastic about sharing their own stories and connecting with the younger generation.

The project thrived on a simple yet profound formula: show the film, stir the conversation, and watch the connections bloom. "It's like magic," I often say, "you see these students and older adults, initially hesitant, gradually opening up, sharing stories, laughing, sometimes even crying together. It's beautiful."

Throughout the quarter-long project, students were matched with an older adult for a series of interviews with questions from the *Lives Well Lived* film being utilized as a starting point to initiate a discussion. The foundation of questions derived from the film provided a framework for heartfelt bilateral conversations between students and older adults. These interactions unfolded independently four times during the term, culminating in a final event where students shared the knowledge they had acquired during their time together through presentations and with written memoirs. The lofty goal? To share a deeper understanding of each other's perspectives and life experiences, and to exchange wisdom between generations.

What we discovered through this project was truly remarkable. It became evident that, despite age differences, people share many similarities. We were on a mission to challenge age-related stereotypes and biases, one genuine friendship at a time. Since its inception, the program has touched the lives of over 600 individuals, successfully erasing generational boundaries.

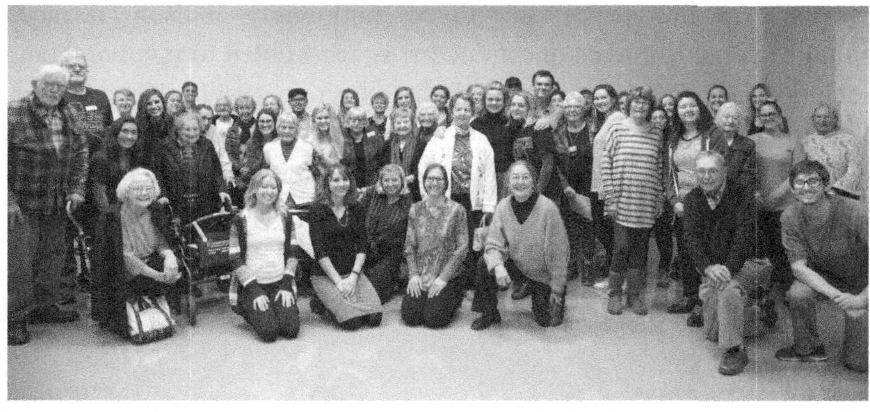

Intergenerational pilot project wrap party, Fall 2018

Measuring outcomes...

Professor Sara Bartlett's research on the program yielded profound insights. She taught two sections of the Psychology of Aging class. One section was the control group. They watched the film but did not participate in the *Lives Well Lived* learning module. The other section watched the film and completed the *Lives Well Lived* project. Her findings revealed that students in the *Lives Well Lived* group displayed less negative bias and fewer stereotypes about aging compared to the control group. Students in the *Lives Well Lived* program often used the word 'friend' in their responses, emphasizing the personal connections they had formed, by contrast to the control group. Moreover, students reported a reduced fear of aging themselves, thanks to their interactions with older adults who continue to enjoy life. (Bartlett et al., 2021 and 2022)

What truly makes this project a standout are the stories, the shared moments. Professor Sara Bartlett shared one such story: "There was this student, initially skeptical, who ended up forming a bond with an older adult that was so strong, it transformed his outlook on life. It's moments like these that remind us why we do what we do."

The program also defied socioeconomic boundaries, showing that success isn't solely determined by wealth or status. There were moments that left a lasting impression, like when we worked with residents at the senior subsidized community, Judson Terrace. Initially, some residents questioned why we wanted to involve them, feeling that they hadn't achieved anything remarkable. However, as the project progressed, it became evident that the students gained just as much from these interactions as they did with older adults of higher socioeconomic status, demonstrating we all connect on a human level and have valuable lessons to share.

Transitioning to an online format...

The COVID-19 pandemic brought both challenges and opportunities. We transitioned the project to an online format, collaborating with Aaron Santis, Program Lead at Senior Planet (part of AARP). Overcoming the digital divide is a priority for Senior Planet with initiatives aimed at providing affordable internet access and teaching effective tool utilization. The intergenerational program exemplified the organization's commitment to empowering older adults, reshaping perceptions, and fostering inclusivity and accessibility. Aaron Santis shared:

The transformation is palpable. It's one thing to talk about bridging the gap, and quite another to actually see it happen. These conversations, they're not just chit-chat. They're life lessons, shared across generations. The program encouraged intentional dialogues about life's meaning and personal perspectives, enabling participants to view things from different angles and gain insights that wouldn't typically arise in day-to-day interactions. Participants, especially those lacking connections to younger generations, appreciated the opportunity for social interaction and personal connection with individuals from different age groups. It has been heartening to see students from different parts of the country connecting with older adults and broadening their horizons.

Transitioning the project to an online format during the pandemic brought significant benefits. The greatest advantage was the ability to continue these intergenerational projects even during challenging times. The digital platform allowed us to maintain connections and reach students and older adults who were isolated during the pandemic. The opportunity for students to interact with people from different parts of the country enriched their learning experience. It was interesting to note that the screen, though a barrier for some, provided a sense of comfort and distance that allowed students to be more vulnerable in their interactions.

It was during the pandemic that Dr. Elizabeth Fugate-Whitlock of the University of North Carolina Wilmington was looking for a program that she could use to bring older adults and students together, and stumbled upon the *Lives Well Lived* program. Fugate-Whitlock shared, "The project was a perfect fit for our curriculum during the pandemic, offering a powerful learning experience." She noted that students who often lack connections with older generations questioned their implicit biases about aging and gained a more well-rounded perspective of the aging experience through the program. "My students often start with a set image of what aging is. But through this project, they discover a whole new world—a world where aging is not just about getting old but about living well."

Dr. Tina Newsham, also from UNCW, praised the *Lives Well Lived* project as a valuable addition to gerontology courses at UNCW, fostering intergenerational conversations about aging and challenging negative perceptions of growing older. "The program aligns with the university's commitment to being age-friendly, emphasizing the benefits of an aging society. Beyond academic learning, it's about forming human connections and fostering mutual respect across ages."

The transition to an online format during the pandemic also presented unique opportunities to UNCW students working with the *Lives Well Lived* project. Fugate-Whitlock observed, "Going digital allowed us to connect our students with diverse life stories nationwide." Newsham echoed this sentiment: "The online format, while challenging, opened doors to broader interactions and learning opportunities." Both professors integrated the film into their classes and collaborated with Natalie Quinn, a student in the Master of Science in Applied Gerontology program at UNCW, in a paper published in the *AGHExchange (Academy for Gerontology in Higher Education)* newsletter, detailing the project's impact on students' understanding of aging. (Quinn et al., 2022). Impacts of the project were assessed through the Expectations Regarding Aging scale (Sarkisian et al.,

2005) prior to any interactions between partners, and again at the end of the project, along with an open-ended questionnaire about their experiences. Expectations regarding aging improved on 75% of the items, and participants indicated qualitatively that their experiences with the intergenerational interactions were positive.

I have worked with corporations as well, bringing the project to companies such as Land O'Lakes were Philomena Morrissey Satre, Director of DEI (Diversity, Equity, and Inclusion) and head of the Aging Successfully ERG (Employee Resources Group) said:

In my constant quest for engaging and insightful content, whether it's through an online seminar, conference, or in this instance, the remarkable Lives Well Lived film I'm perpetually attuned to opportunities that can enrich our corporate culture at Land O'Lakes. Prior to this, our DEI learning sessions had not yet delved into the realm of intergenerational understanding. This gap underscored the relevance and potential impact of the film, positioning it as an ideal catalyst to commence this vital dialogue within our organization.

The decision to integrate the Lives Well Lived program into our framework was strategic, aiming to ignite intergenerational connections and insights. The collaboration between our Young Professionals Network and Aging Successfully groups in co-sponsoring this initiative was a deliberate move. It wasn't just about focusing on aging successfully; it was about creating a platform where wisdom, experiences, and perspectives from different generations could intersect and enrich one another.

What I've learned is that you could show a hundred PowerPoint slides, and then you could have a few people tell powerful stories that bring the content to life. And that's what people will remember; it is the powerful story. This approach aligns seamlessly with our objectives at Land O'Lakes, making the program a valuable and memorable addition to our DEI initiatives.

PBS LearningMedia website...

bit.ly/LWLPBSLearningMedia

The inclusion of the "Intergenerational Connections through Storytelling | *Lives Well Lived*" resource on the PBS LearningMedia website is an immensely gratifying development. This platform serves as a treasure trove for K-12 educators, offering them invaluable access to a wealth of *Lives Well Lived* resources thoughtfully aligned with age-appropriate core standards curated by PBS. It is designed to be a collaboration between students and older adults, bringing together generations so that we can collectively expand our understanding of each other and grow exponentially. (PBS Learning Media, 2024)

It is never too early to begin connecting generations and combating the stereotypes of ageism. According to the World Health Organization (WHO), "Children as young as four years old become aware of their culture's age stereotypes. From that age onwards, they internalize and use these stereotypes to guide their feelings and behavior towards people of different ages." (WHO, 2021)

As educators, we understand the profound impact that intergenerational connections can have on the development of young minds. The stories and experiences shared through the *Lives Well Lived* Intergenerational Project serve as an extraordinary resource for teachers seeking to foster empathy, understanding, and appreciation among their students. By integrating these resources into their curricula, educators have the power to bridge generational gaps, impart timeless wisdom, and inspire the next generation to embrace the richness of life's journey.

The vision continues…

My big vision for this project is to have *Lives Well Lived* integrated into high school and college curricula across the country, and I am delighted that we have been named a Generations United's Program of Distinction. Generations United's Program of Distinction is an elite designation that serves as the U.S. benchmark for intergenerational programs and is based on the criteria that underpin the effectiveness of high-quality intergenerational programs. With this designation, I am that much closer to realizing that dream.

The most significant revelation from this project has been the realization that, at the core, we all share more similarities than differences, with age being the primary distinction. It's a testament to the power of human connection and storytelling. Stereotypes and prejudices, including ageism, tend to dissolve when you form genuine friendships with someone from a different age group. Together, we can work towards the creation of a more inclusive intergenerational world, where the wisdom of the past enriches the aspirations of the future. The potential for transformative learning experiences is boundless, and it is our collective responsibility to harness this potential for the benefit of our students and society as a whole.

Looking back on this journey, I'm filled with a sense of gratitude and wonder. The *Lives Well Lived* Intergenerational Project has not only challenged stereotypes and biases but has also enriched the lives of countless individuals. It is more than just an educational initiative; it's a testament to the enduring power of storytelling and shared experiences. It highlights the importance of understanding and celebrating life at all stages, fostering connections that transcend generational gaps. It has reminded us that a well-lived life knows no age limit and that connections forged across generations have the power to change the world.

Have you considered bringing a similar project to your community, educational institution or corporation? Reach out, we can make that happen!

Sample Project Timeline

Service-learning introduction #1: Organize a session for the screening of *Lives Well Lived*, followed by a discussion and networking period. This session can be conducted either entirely in person or virtually, featuring a Q&A segment with structured discussion groups or online breakout rooms.

Questions to ask include:

- In what ways did the film either confirm or dispel any stereotypes you have about older people?
- What lessons did you take away from this film and do you think you will use the advice?
- How do you define a life well lived?
- What bit of personal wisdom or advice have you received from an older adult?

Participant engagement phase: Secure the participation of approximately 35-40 older adults by collaborating with the site coordinator. Pair each older adult with a student, ensuring the setup is suitable for either in-person or virtual interaction.

Service-learning encounter #2: Arrange an introductory session for groups at the field site or via a virtual platform as per the planned schedule.

- Start with a brief overview of the project.
- Encourage students and older adults to exchange personal stories, discuss hometowns, academic backgrounds, employment, hobbies, and life experiences, with the flexibility to interact in person or online.
- Ask older adults to share insights into their past professions, significant life events, and other personal anecdotes with their student partners.

Service-learning interaction #3: Organize a meeting for groups to conduct interviews, which can be held face-to-face or online on the scheduled date. Students use the *Lives Well Lived Discussion Guide* to frame their questions and record the responses either in writing or as an audio file. Simultaneously, older adults have the opportunity to interview their student partners using their own set of questions or the ones from the guide. These questions serve as a starting point for the memoir project, where students might write an essay, craft a piece of art, or create an approved final project that demonstrates what the student learned about the older adult they partnered with, along with how their perceptions of aging have changed.

Service-learning session #4: Schedule a session for groups to either proceed with the second part of their interview or to collaboratively draft and review the initial version of the memoir project, inviting feedback and suggestions for refinement from the older adults participating.

Service-learning finale #5: Invite students to give presentations, sharing their experiences and showcasing the memoirs created in collaboration with their older adult partners. Older adults have the option to either co-present with their student partners or engage as audience members.

The Final Project:

The students will take what they have learned from their interaction with the elder and complete the following:

- Compose a memoir of the older adult's life. The memoir can be a formatted copy of the interview transcript, a digital or paper-based scrapbook, a poster, an original poem, a short video. Be as creative as you would like.
- Write a paper connecting their experience with what they have learned about the psychology of aging.
- Create a slide presentation about their experience doing this project, which they will present at the wrap party at the end of the project. The presentation should include the answers to these questions:

What is the older adult's secret to a Life Well Lived?

What is my definition of a Life Well Lived?

What have I learned and how have I changed from this project?

What is the biggest takeaway?

What STUDENTS have said about this project…

- "My favorite part of the project was getting to know the older adult I interviewed, seeing the richness of her life and her remarkable resilience. This experience taught me we can all contribute meaningfully to life until our very last moment."
- "I really valued learning about life transitions and events like marriage, career, losing loved ones, which I rarely get to hear about because of how age-segregated our culture is. It makes life seem less intimidating the more I learn how other people have worked through life's highs and lows."
- "Through this project, I not only gained a new friendship but also a fresh perspective on aging. It provided me with a valuable opportunity to engage with a different age group in a meaningful way."
- "I have completely changed my perspective of older generations for the better."
- "After this project I feel more excited about my future and will try to cherish every moment I have in my life even more!"
- "My favorite part of the project was getting to build intergenerational relationships. Applying the information we learned in class to a real-life interaction was very beneficial and impactful."
- "I learned you can accomplish any goal you have at any stage of life, there are no limits. I changed through this project by now viewing aging as more time to learn and grow."
- "I used to fear aging; I viewed the changes as stripping away the most valuable parts of my identity. But my partner showed me that aging is beautiful and brings the opportunity to explore other parts of who you are."

What OLDER ADULTS have said about this project...

- "I think the project is very insightful. At a time when we talk about increasing social isolation and loneliness, this project is very valuable because it brings generations together. It gives us the opportunity to share experiences and learn from each other."
- "Friends can come from all walks of life and be any age. We have so much to learn from each other."
- "I loved the stereotype-smashing that happens in this program—from both directions."
- "This has been one of the most rewarding experiences of my life. I have a newfound hope for our future."
- "I was so impressed with the similar threads that were woven through our every conversation. We realized we had far more in common than our differences."
- "I was amazed by how much I discovered about myself through conversations with students. It was uplifting to have someone who truly listened to what I had to say."
- "This project has filled me with optimism. The students I spoke with have been a source of inspiration. Because of them, I hold a very positive outlook on what lies ahead."
- "Community is important throughout your life. It's not just about how you are impacted, but how you impact others."

Sources:

Bartlett, S.P., Solomon, P. & Gellis, Z. (2021) Comparative effectiveness of intergenerational service-learning programs on student outcomes of knowledge, attitude, and ageism. *Educational Gerontology*, 47(12), 559-573. bit.ly/4aX6OX1

Bartlett, S.P., Solomon, P. & Gellis, Z. (2022) "They're Not All Grumps": A Qualitative Process Examination of Two Intergenerational SERVICE-LEARNING Programs. *Journal of Intergenerational Relationships.* bit.ly/3JiIbbH

Quinn, Natalie. Fugate-Whitlock, Ph.D., Elizabeth. M.K. Newsham, Ph.D. Tina. Bergman, Sky. (2022) Implementing a Virtual, Age-Friendly Intergenerational Program. *AGEExchange*, 45(1), 8-12. bit.ly/3U3XR7l

Sarkisian, C. A., Steers, W. N., Hays, R. D., & Mangione, C. M. (2005). Development of the 12-item expectations regarding aging survey. *The Gerontologist*, 45(2), 240-248.

World Health Organization (WHO). "Ageing: Ageism" Who.int. March 18, 2021. bit.ly/3W31D3Q

PBS Learning Media. "Intergenerational Connections through Storytelling | Lives Well Lived" PBSlearningmedia.com. bit.ly/LWLPBSLearningMedia

CONNECTING GENERATIONS

Every individual possesses a unique story and intrinsic value, contributing something meaningful to the collective mosaic of humanity. To unlock this potential, we must establish connections.

Human beings, Homo sapiens, are inherently tribal creatures. Our ancestral journey began in Africa, where we embarked on a monumental diaspora hundreds of thousands of years ago. Along this odyssey, we huddled around campfires to share the discovery of fire, traded secrets for survival, crafted tools, and adapted to diverse environments from deserts to the Arctic. Our evolution gave birth to writing, culture, values, art, and science.

In the unfolding narrative of the 21st century, humanity has witnessed a profound transformation in its tools and methods, yet the core of our tribal essence endures. Amidst this era of rapid technological advancement, we find ourselves more connected, yet—paradoxically—more divided than ever before. Our world has become a digital agora where ideas circulate with the speed of light, where cat videos on social media platforms elicit global smiles, and where collective human experiences, from combating global pandemics to reveling in sporting victories or mourning environmental disasters, unite us in shared 'cyber' moments. Remarkably, in this century of achievements and advancements, we face a unique and growing chasm—that of generational divide. Society has increasingly categorized and related to people primarily based on their age.

The intricate fabric of extended, multi-generational families, which once formed the bedrock of societal structure, has started to unravel. I was fortunate to have grown up in a household spanning four generations. In this setup, my grandparents played a central role within our family, generously sharing their traditions, stories, and wisdom. Their constant presence enabled me to forge deep emotional connections and provided me with a unique perspective and invaluable guidance. In return, my grandparents derived a profound sense of purpose and belonging.

Today, it has become a common practice for families to reside geographically far from one another. The shift away from intergenerational living has sadly led to a significant reduction in opportunities for meaningful exchanges between different age groups. This decline has resulted in fewer cherished moments between grandchildren and grandparents.

Age segregation is prevalent in contemporary society, characterized by the physical and social separation of individuals based on their age. This segregation takes various forms, from the systematic grouping of children by age in educational institutions to the isolation of older adults in care facilities. This generational segregation extends into the workforce, where mature individuals often struggle to find their place. The invaluable experience and knowledge they possess are frequently overlooked, leading to a workforce that misses out on the benefits of age-diverse perspectives. This not only impacts the older adults, who find themselves confined to roles and environments that may not fully appreciate their contributions, but also affects the societal fabric, which loses the opportunity to be enriched by a vibrant, intergenerational and productive community.

In short, we are far from perfect.

People from all walks of life are realizing that modern society is disconnecting us. We have erred in the way we have divided generations, making 'others' of our older and younger generations. In short, we are living in an age-segregated society, particularly underscored by the glaring disparities exposed by the global pandemic.

As we navigate the complexities of the 21st century, it becomes imperative to bridge this generational divide, to create spaces where the young and old can interact meaningfully, and to recognize the value of all ages in every aspect of societal life. In doing so, we can move toward a more inclusive understanding, an enriched global community, where the wisdom of the past and the innovations of the present coalesce to create a harmonious and forward-looking society.

So, what actions are people taking to rekindle these vital connections between generations?

Why do we yearn for such connections? Why do our well-being and health suffer when they are absent? Addressing these questions is not just about individual impact; it is about recognizing the repercussions on families, communities, and society as a whole when we disregard the profound benefits that intergenerational connections offer.

In the following section, we will explore the stories and initiatives of thought leaders worldwide who are pioneering innovative ways to bring generations together. These visionaries approach the topic from various angles, offering unique programs and solutions. Through workshops, art, music, and even simple conversations over coffee and pastries, they are helping us rediscover the immense value of these connections, both for individuals and communities.

What have these initiatives observed?

While there are a multitude of programs encompassing people from diverse cultures and backgrounds, it is not surprising that they all share similar motives for launching their efforts and report consistent outcomes—ageism diminishes when generations connect. Ageism thrives on perceiving others as different, but when you discover shared interests, you find common ground and recognize a bit of yourself in each other, regardless of age.

In addition to combating the stereotypes of ageism, perhaps the most poignant reason for bringing generations together is to combat the epidemic of social isolation and loneliness. In some way or another, each organization that I interviewed highlights the tangible benefits of intergenerational connections in mitigating feelings of loneliness and isolation, providing both young and old participants with a sense of belonging and emotional support. Every organization I interviewed highlighted these benefits, noting the mutual enrichment that arises from such interactions.

Connecting generations nurtures reciprocity and empathy, fostering respect irrespective of age. Everyone, regardless of age, experiences the opportunity to form meaningful connections and relationships. Young adults who spend time with supportive older adults become more engaged in their studies, achieve better grades, and cultivate healthier relationships. Children benefit significantly from intergenerational interactions, enhancing their problem-solving abilities, vocabulary, and social-emotional skills. Older adults, in turn, experience a renewed sense of purpose, responsibility, and identity.

People of different ages who spend time together build bonds of trust, perceiving strangers from a kinder, more trusting perspective. Love and support are universal languages, and when you belong, you care. Individuals come together to create music, share meals, sit on stoops exchanging stories, and converse.

Organizations are pairing older adults with students to provide companionship and support in exchange for affordable housing arrangements, breaking down stereotypes about different generations. Generations come together to pursue their love for music and performance through orchestras and bands, with students benefiting from the guidance and skills of their older mentors. Older individuals rediscover their passion for music and gain newfound confidence.

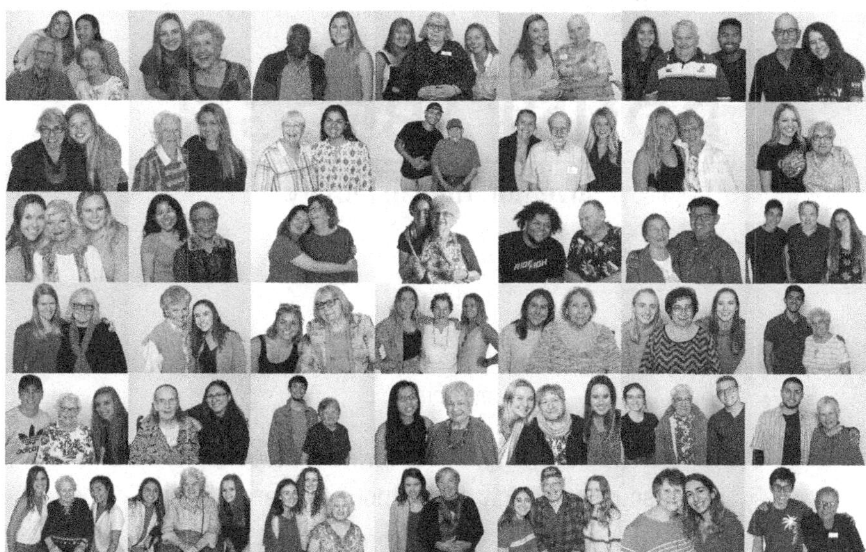

Mixing the perspectives of different generations fosters productive discussions that often yield creative and agile solutions. It serves as a powerful reminder that compromise between generations can be incredibly impactful. In some cases, groups encourage older adults to hop back on their bikes, quite literally, through cycling tours of their towns and surrounding regions.

Numerous initiatives involve different generations in art projects, creating communities of older adults within modern family apartment complexes. The range of projects and purposes is vast, while learning every day. Bringing generations together in unconventional spaces has remarkable impacts on all participants, young and old alike.

Without further delay, let's delve into these remarkable programs, one by one, and experience the magic of intergenerational connections.

RONNI ABERGEL

Inventor, Human Library

humanlibrary.org

Creating a special dialogue room, where taboo topics can be discussed openly and without condemnation.

"We provide a place where people who would otherwise never talk find room for conversation."

I've always been naturally curious. As a child, I constantly asked questions which my parents said weren't always appropriate or in line with societal norms. Often, I would address topics considered taboo, the elephant in the room. That would be my specialty. People thought I was trying to be provocative; I wasn't. I was simply very inquisitive.

As I grew older, I realized that there are so many conversations that are avoided because they lack the proper context or framework. Yet, these discussions are crucial for building self and social awareness and better relationships. I imagined creating a safe space where no question is deemed foolish or inappropriate, regardless of how it is phrased or its subject matter. This space would be a place where volunteers, resilient and open, would answer questions they've heard countless times, explaining their appearance, habits, disabilities, or mental and neurodiverse conditions. Many of these individuals, often facing stigma, discrimination, or hate crimes, are eager to educate and help others understand their experiences. By sharing their stories, they could demonstrate their value and contribute to a more inclusive and just society.

I created the Human Library to give voice to many marginalized groups, promoting understanding and visibility. For me, this project also has a personal aspect; it's about seeking acceptance, something I yearned for in my youth. I was passionate and often misinterpreted which led to isolation and the need to better articulate my feelings and reactions.

Everyone desires understanding and acceptance, especially those who might have unique communication styles or needs. My goal was to create a platform where people could express themselves and learn about others. This endeavor, though not financially lucrative, is deeply fulfilling and meaningful. It's a calling for me, especially now I'm in my fifties. It's about helping others find the acceptance I lacked earlier in life. This is my journey and contribution, creating a space where everyone can be understood and accepted.

I like to think of each one of us as a book, a book where the pages are being written each day and, as such, it becomes the book of our life. At the Human Library you can borrow books, just like at any other library. But our 'books' are actual people with personal stories and a lived experience they are willing to share. All of our books are drawn from groups in our society that are negatively marginalized or targeted with (or vulnerable to) prejudice and discrimination because of their identity, lifestyle, occupation, social status, religious belief, sexuality, ethnic origin, or something similar. Every one of us has prejudices and biases, but not everyone has the opportunity to explore diversity within a safe space and find out if what we believe we know about other people is true. The Human Library works to create safe spaces for this type of dialogue, where anyone can join and meet their prejudices, face to face. The classic saying is, "Don't judge a book by its cover." But at the Human Library, we won´t tell you not to judge. We offer you an opportunity to unjudge and engage.

Our books do not represent an entire group. They are only speaking on behalf of themselves. This allows for the individually lived experience to take center stage, all aspects included. While 'Age' for now, is not a title in our library, it is an inherent facet of life, and is naturally a part of the conversations we facilitate.

There is a big difference between a trans-woman in her sixties and one in her twenties. One has primarily lived in a world where very few knew what it meant to be transgender, and the other has primarily lived in a world where a legal transition is possible. As an 'outsider,' hearing each woman's story gives vastly different views of the lived experience of a transgender person.

Just as well, a gay man in his seventies now, was a young man during the height of the AIDS crisis. He may have buried many of his friends after watching them suffer with a frightening and unknown disease. He may have never come out to his parents or his colleagues, hiding his identity out of necessity. A gay man in his twenties today lives in a world where, at least in Denmark, the Human Library has its headquarters. He can be out and about with his boyfriend, safely go to gay nightclubs and join the Pride festival every year. It is also, to some extent, possible to be 'out' at his job, marry, adopt and never have to watch a friend or lover die from an avoidable disease. To the gay man in his seventies, this life would probably seem like a dream, while to the young man, the tragedy of the 1980s seems equally unreal.

Having such a distinction between generations is likely to cause misunderstandings, resentment, and assumptions, unless conversation is encouraged. Having open, honest conversations is the primary road to meaningful connection. This is the mission and core of the Human Library organization.

The positive outcomes we see are human connection and greater empathy across generations. With opportunities to mirror, reflect, and gain insight to the journey of others, we are able to build a better understanding for each other and achieve a stronger sense of inclusion and acceptance. This is a place where we do not live in fear of each other, but rather, in mutual appreciation of what each generation, and each group (in all of their diversity) are bringing to the community.

Whether it be targeted programs or activities that are somehow able to bridge divides and appeal to intergenerational target groups, the importance of having these meeting places cannot be underestimated. The social fabric of our communities is based on a sense of cohesion and belonging to the community, where we feel genuinely responsible for each other, and can work together on common goals.

Everything around us has been shaped by the knowledge accumulated through generations, yet many of the youth today lack access to meaningful spaces with older generations. Meanwhile, loneliness is a cross-generational global challenge. The Human Library helps counter some of that alienation by creating a safe space where we can safely explore mankind and our own biases, to challenge the stigmas and the stereotypes by meeting those who, on the surface, would seem to represent them.

In our work, we create learning opportunities around the world. These are places where marginalized and stigmatized groups can help the rest of the community learn how to be more inclusive, compassionate, and less judgmental. We are working to help give a voice to the many who suffer from our lack of understanding and acceptance.

At the Human Library you will not be judged, but you will have an opportunity to *un*judge someone and yourself.

MARCI ALBOHER

Vice President, CoGenerate

cogenerate.org

Bridging generational divides to co-create the future.

"The beauty of intergenerational programs is that we can learn from each other, and about the past, to help shape the future."

I've always collected mentors. My mom and dad had their own business, but neither was college educated. So when I started looking for jobs, I needed guidance I wasn't getting from them. When I got my first job as a lawyer, and later as a writer, I sought mentors who had those kinds of experiences.

When I hit my thirties and forties and realized I would not have children, I wondered how I was going to meet and form relationships with younger people. I don't have a big family; I don't belong to a faith community, and I don't have strong neighborhood ties. I also realized that the only way to stay relevant in the workplace was to interact with younger people and be plugged into new ways of thinking and communicating, innovative trends, and how to navigate the ever-changing world.

After researching several mentoring organizations in New York City, I landed on Girls Write Now, a multigenerational group of women and gender-expansive teens, which became the heart and soul of my community. Because we share a common interest—writing—it's easy to get to know people who are different from me, whether that's because of age, ethnicity or cultural background, identity, or sexual orientation. I was drawn to this particular community because I felt I had something to offer to young people who are mostly aspiring first-generation college students (like I was), but I get a whole lot more than I give. I now have a collection of young women who are part of my life in various ways—some feel like mentees, some are friends, others are woven into my writing or professional life.

Now that I'm in my fifties, I see the bigger patterns. When you're young, you crave older people; when you're starting to feel older, you realize you need younger ones to stay fresh and energized, nimble and relevant.

My role model for forming intergenerational relationships is my mother who is a magnet for attracting younger friends. She's the embodiment of what Gina Pell calls a 'perennial'—a person of any age who continues to learn, grow and remain relevant, refusing to be defined by their generation. At 81, my mom is well-versed in pop culture, always using the latest technology and routinely socializing with people decades younger than she is.

For nearly twenty years, my mom and I hosted an intergenerational clothing swap. I saw women in their seventies and eighties give heirloom-style items (fur coats, real jewelry, vintage handbags) to twenty-somethings they met only moments before. And when women brought children, that's where the real magic happened. At one swap, a four-year-old girl in a tutu (acquired at the swap) kept us entertained, and a bevy of aunties allowed her mom to focus on browsing. Women left, not only with new clothes, but with new friends and job leads.

The beauty of intergenerational gatherings, even simple ones like this one, is that we can learn from each other, and about the past, to help shape the future. In many contexts, the 'other' is someone we need to learn to understand. We can remember what it was like to be young; and by meeting people ahead of us, we can imagine what it might be like to be older. Bridging that difference could even be a step on the way to bridging other divides, and to learning from, and understanding, each other.

Today, I work at CoGenerate (formerly Encore.org), a national nonprofit dedicated to bringing older and younger people together to solve critical problems and bridge divides. I lead our strategy work around narrative change and community building. On any given day, I launch new partnerships, speak at events, write essays to advance our thought leadership, or talk to members of the media about how to bridge the age gap.

We borrowed the cogeneration language from the energy field, where it means multiple power sources coming together to result in something far more powerful. We loved that metaphor, and what we mean by 'cogeneration' is older and younger people joining each other to co-create a better future. We support leaders who work on social co-generational solutions to a wide variety of issues, from cross-mentoring programs to ways of reimagining strategies in the workplace or in our community. We like to think about cogeneration as an idea that can exist where we live, work, worship, in any aspect of life.

When our organization evolved from Encore.org to CoGenerate, we worked to age-diversify our team, our board, and all the networks and communities that we support. We've also age-diversified our senior leadership by having a co-generational, co-leadership model.

Our founder and Co-CEO Marc Freedman and Co-CEO Eunice Lin Nichols come from different generations with separate experiences and views of leadership. They are learning from one another in all kinds of interesting ways.

It's a real joy that my working life is all about something that feels so magical to me.

VANESSA ARCARA

President and Co-Founder, Third Act and Senior to Senior

thirdact.org

Building a community of Americans over the age of sixty determined to change the world for the better.

"Together, we can use our life experience, skills, and resources to build a better tomorrow. Third Act exists to bring Americans over sixty into our fights for progressive action, specifically safeguarding our democracy and protecting our climate."

"Experienced Americans" are the fastest-growing part of the population: 10,000 people a day pass the 60-year mark. Contrary to the assumption that age fosters conservatism due to a desire to protect the status quo, this generation witnessed profound positive changes in their youth, such as the Civil Rights Movement, efforts to end major conflicts, and the advancement of women's rights. They possess the key to addressing critical challenges facing our planet and society. The collective voice of this group holds sway in Washington and Wall

Street, driven by their significant voting power and substantial share of the nation's assets. Furthermore, many within this demographic have children, grandchildren, and even great-grandchildren, providing them with tangible reasons to be deeply invested in creating a better future.

The ten guiding principles of Third Act emphasize kindness, inclusivity, humility, support, accountability, and creativity in pursuing progressive change. These principles promote nonviolence, collaboration, and an intergenerational approach, recognizing the importance of bridging generational gaps and working together to address critical issues, while valuing self-care and generosity without overextending resources.

My inspiration for getting into intergenerational work stems from my childhood. I grew up as an only child in a suburban area outside of Manhattan, where my family had limited close relatives nearby. I always longed for more elders in my life and felt most comfortable engaging with people from different generations. This inclination stayed with me throughout my life.

My interest in creating Third Act, especially the Senior to Senior program, came about while working alongside Bill McKibben at 350.org, a global grassroots movement to solve the climate crisis. We noticed the incredible power of youth-led movements for justice, particularly in the climate justice movement. We also observed that a huge amount of volunteer work in our movement spaces was being done by individuals over the age of sixty. This helped us realize it didn't feel right asking eighteen-year-olds to fix the biggest problems the world has ever faced all on their own. We wanted to tap into the potential of our older generations, who were also willing to roll up their sleeves and bring their experience and passion to bear.

The value of intergenerational connections, as I've witnessed, is immense. At Third Act, our team intentionally includes individuals from diverse age groups, ranging from people in their mid-twenties to those in their late sixties and seventies. This mix of perspectives fosters productive discussions and often results in creative and agile solutions. It's a reminder that compromise between generations can be incredibly powerful.

Our Senior to Senior program, an intergenerational voter registration initiative, focuses on registering high school students to vote. Every year, four million Americans turn eighteen and become eligible to vote, but fewer than half of them vote. However, once registered, youth *do* vote, in large numbers. In every presidential election from 2004 to 2020, more than 75% of registered 18- to 24-year-olds voted, with 80% in 2020. The solution is to register newly eligible youth voters while they are still in high school.

Third Act partners with The Civics Center (TCC) and is an active member of the Ready to Vote Coalition. We leverage the reliability of older Americans as voters and encourage them to share their experiences and stories with younger generations. This not only inspires younger people but also helps them connect with the significance of political engagement in their lives. The program aims to bridge the generational gap and stimulate discussions about the importance of civic participation.

While it's challenging to pinpoint the exact number of students impacted, we worked with partners like the Civic Center, which had a goal to contact 1,000 high schools across the country. Third Act contributed to reaching over 600 of these schools, exceeding 60% of the goal. This highlights the potential of our approach and the dedication of our volunteers, who bring a unique level of commitment to our initiatives. Newer Third Act Working Groups have organized with partners to convene 'dorm storms' where Third Actors are helping register students on college campuses in key districts. I have no doubt we'll see a lot more creativity in the coming months about how to make connections and real impact in getting new voters on the rolls.

Intergenerational work holds incredible value. It creates a platform for sharing wisdom, learning from one another, and collectively addressing critical issues. Through Third Act and the Senior to Senior program, we aim to harness the power of multiple generations coming together to make a positive impact on our society and democracy.

DR. LEWIS J. BERNSTEIN

Co-founder, Sesame 3G Mentoring

3gmentoring.org

A three-generation mental wellness initiative: In a world where preschoolers, high school and college students, and older adults are increasingly isolated, our mission is to deepen connections, grow confidence, and strengthen skills—using the joy of Sesame Street to build intergenerational relationships.

"It may be difficult to envision older adults, students, and very young children joining together in conversation. But we have found that there is learning and joy in this unlikely combination—and that all three generations benefit."

I tell people it took me 43 years to graduate from preschool. I was fortunate to work at the Sesame Workshop in various capacities because I was inspired by the mission of 'helping kids everywhere grow smarter, stronger, and kinder.' When I retired, I found myself at a crossroads. While I had stepped away from my role, I wasn't ready to step away from making a meaningful impact on the world. I thought, *what can I do?*

As I explored this newfound path, I delved into literature that resonated the notion of 'encore careers' and the pursuit of relevance beyond traditional retirement age. I was already part of the SWAN (Sesame Workshop Alumni Network) at the workshop, and I figured that there had to be other people like me among the alum who wanted to give back in some way. I thought, *why don't we think about doing something where we can somehow pass our experience on to other generations?* That marked the initial seed of inspiration for Sesame 3G Mentoring.

The other catalyst for Sesame 3G Mentoring was a response to pressing societal challenges, magnified by the COVID-19 pandemic. There is an ever-growing crisis of loneliness, social isolation, and depression in America—particularly for older adults and teenagers. This led us to contemplate, "What if older adults could provide mentorship to these teens?" Sesame Street segments, with their universal appeal, became our tool for engagement. '3G' represents the involvement of three generations: older adults, teens, and preschoolers, forming the heart of the program.

Sesame 3G Mentoring bridges these generations through Sesame Street segments that serve as catalysts for conversations. Older adults who are Sesame Workshop alum, engage with high school students, sharing life experiences and discussing the chosen segments. The high school students then mentor preschoolers using the curated Sesame Street segments that spark discussion, empathy, and joy. The program's circular nature enhances the exchange of wisdom, enriching the lives of participants across generations. We have the three generations working together. The teen is in the middle, getting advice and thoughts from the older generation, and then they are given the opportunity and trust to interact with the preschoolers.

The concept of intergenerational connections brought a rich array of benefits woven into the lives of each generation involved. For the older adult participants, this experience offered a profound shift in perspective. Many of them had never truly interacted with teenagers. Engaging with this younger generation infused them with newfound optimism for the future. They witnessed the remarkable talents of these teens—bright, committed, innovative individuals brimming with potential. This revelation sparked a renewed sense of hope, not only in the possibilities for the teenagers but also in the reciprocal enrichment they could bring to the seniors.

The insights shared by the teenagers were truly eye-opening. Many of them confided that their interactions with their parents were few and far between, let alone with someone from an older generation. Engaging in this program exposed them to an array of new skills—from mastering email, a tool they rarely used, to taking on the responsibility of scheduling meetings, even with preschoolers. The journey also encompassed cognitive growth, expanding a teenager's understanding of various concepts.

However, the most significant revelation for both the teenagers and the preschoolers was the emergence of a unique bond. Some preschoolers affectionately addressed their teen mentors as 'best friends,' a sentiment reciprocated by the teens. This profound connection extended beyond mere labels; it illustrated the preschoolers' recognition of their teen mentors as individuals wholly invested in them. The preschool teachers observed this heartwarming development, emphasizing that the program provided an environment where the preschoolers felt genuinely seen and heard. Their rapport with the teen mentors became a source of invaluable learning, teaching them how to forge connections with young adults in ways that transcended the typical classroom interactions.

This interplay of three generations resulted in what we term a 'three generation glorious circle,' seamlessly merging their unique experiences into a collective journey of shared growth and understanding.

DEB BIBBINS

Founder, For All Ages

forallages.org

Connecting the generations and inspiring action to end loneliness, reduce ageism, and improve health.

"Connecting the generations has the power to positively impact the mental, physical, and social health of people of all ages, and to reduce ageism."

The vision of For All Ages was conceived after spending hours researching the topics of loneliness and isolation following my father's passing. His social network shrank over the years due to the death of many of his friends. And while he had been spending a lot of time with his brother, my uncle experienced a medical emergency and died suddenly. My father died a few short weeks later.

It is my belief that loneliness played a significant part in his passing. After learning that more than half of American adults were experiencing loneliness, I decided to do something about it.

Through my experiences as a mentor in my professional life, and as a coach and Girl Scout leader in my personal life, I discovered that intergenerational connection improves the health of both younger and older populations, and simultaneously reduces ageism. That belief set the stage for launching For All Ages.

For All Ages is dedicated to connecting the generations and inspiring action to end loneliness, reduce ageism, and improve health and well-being. Through innovative, evidence-informed and evidence-based programs and events, we create positive, collaborative experiences between the generations that highlight the wisdom and vibrancy of older adults, while countering the loneliness and isolation that are now at epidemic levels across most age groups. We offer a variety of virtual and in-person opportunities for people of different generations to interact, learn from one another, and experience social connection.

When the pandemic began, we created our Tea @ 3 Community, a virtual intergenerational friendship program, to safely connect young adults and older adults, the two loneliest populations. Over five, twelve-week sessions, this program has now provided more than 3,000 hours of impactful, intergenerational connection to college students and older adults. Participants, younger and older, look forward to their weekly phone calls and feel better on the days that they talk. 70% report that participation gives them a sense of belonging and, for many, loneliness decreases. In addition, young adults report a significant increase in their enjoyment from being around older adults, and in their belief that they can learn something from older people. This program now runs each spring and fall and has grown to be our most popular multi-week program. Some Tea-Mates (as we call the intergenerational pairs) continue their friendship long after the twelve-week session ends.

We strive to illuminate the importance of social health and the benefits of intergenerational connection, and to reduce the stigma associated with loneliness (which simply means one needs more social connection). We have spoken on these topics locally, in Connecticut and nationally. I hope that our work to spread awareness inspires people of all ages to improve their social health and the health of those around them.

TONY BROWN

CEO, Heart of Los Angeles (HOLA) and Founder of The Eisner Intergenerational Music Programs

heartofla.org

Helping young people overcome barriers through exceptional, free, integrated programs and personalized guidance in a trusted, nurturing environment.

"Music is a wonderful, highly emotive unifying and healing agent. All ages, races, and genders can find a place to belong. It's about humankind working toward a common goal of making something beautiful."

Growing up, we had a range of ages in one household. My parents were older when I was born and my brothers were a decade or more older than me.

My parents' age and wisdom manifested itself in the calm, capable manner in which they raised me compared to younger, less experienced parents. Throughout my life, I was fascinated by the differences and similarities between our family members and grateful for the gifts passed down from one generation to the next.

I was also fortunate to have highly educated parents who provided me with many opportunities that I wouldn't have had if I'd grown up in another zip code. As I rode the bus from my little town of Sierra Madre to La Cañada High School, I saw the disparity between students whose families had access to resources for extra scholastic and enrichment experiences, and those who did not have that access—primarily people of color. I wanted to make it right.

I got involved with Heart of Los Angeles (HOLA) because I wanted to help children overcome barriers put in their path by providing free programs and services. HOLA is a nonprofit organization founded by Mitchel (Mitch) Moore in 1989 during a volatile and dangerous time in Los Angeles' history. At the time, there were many drive-by shootings in the Westlake neighborhood where Mitch founded HOLA, and he hoped to help young people get off the streets and into safe environments where they could learn, be supported, and have access to enrichment that their schools were not offering them. In 1989, HOLA began in Immanuel Presbyterian Church with just five kids, a basketball, and the vision of a Los Angeles in which every young person has the opportunity to realize their full potential. HOLA began to expand and provide free programs and services for 16- to 24-year-olds, always focused on giving underserved youth opportunities to explore their potential.

I started at HOLA in the early nineties and stayed for three years, watching the organization grow and mature under Mitch's guidance. After earning a Master's degree in Sports Management and working in the sports industry, I returned to Heart of Los Angeles (HOLA) in 2003 as the Chief Development Officer and have been the Chief Executive Officer since 2006. I had also worked as a teacher, and it was the chance to provide opportunity to children that pulled at my heart the most.

Over an almost thirty-five-year period, HOLA has grown to offer students free, exceptional, and integrated programs in: core academics, Science, Technology, Engineering, Arts, Math (STEAM), visual arts, music, and athletics. These engaging and innovative after-school programs help students perform at grade level and matriculate to post-secondary education, often making them the first in their families to achieve a college education. We also provide scholarship opportunities and retention support to first-generation students to ensure their timely graduation from high school, pursuit of post-secondary certifications or advanced degrees, and ultimately, access to vibrant, exciting careers.

Families also benefit from the wellness services that HOLA offers. These services include help with groceries, eyeglasses, vaccinations, and parental support and counseling. Like all anti-poverty organizations, we hope that the resources we provide help entire families now, and continue generationally.

One of the most impactful decisions we've made is to develop an intergenerational music program with The Eisner Foundation that includes three programs: our orchestra, big band, and choir. These programs involve the entire community and create another avenue for youth to make positive connections that will foster their success. The Eisner Foundation has been supporting intergenerational programs for decades now, and when CEO Trent Stamp asked me how I thought that should look at HOLA, I told him that my dream was to connect people through music. Trent thought it was a great concept and suggested that we travel to New Jersey to see an existing orchestra, which included performers of all ages. It was wonderful to see many generations playing music together. I was excited to unite people across generations, as well as across cultures.

The dream became a reality when we created the Eisner Intergenerational Orchestra. Delayed during the COVID-19 pandemic, our newly formed ensemble finally met in the summer of

2021. Ranging from ages eight to eighty, our musicians and singers come from many backgrounds, interests, and abilities. Some are older adults with musical training but no venue for expression; others are young people with minimal to no formal instruction because of school budget cuts or non-existent music education programs. They all, however, have an opportunity to pursue their love of music and experience the joy of performing through the Eisner Intergenerational programs at HOLA.

Many older members of the Eisner Intergenerational Music Programs are retired and living in homes that were built for a family, but now feel empty as their children have grown up and moved out. Members have expressed that if not for the wonderful opportunity to be a part of this group, they would feel lonely and disconnected. Some are highly skilled musicians with conservatory-level training. By playing in the orchestra, these older singers and musicians experience a renewal of purpose as they pursue a lifelong passion and share it with others. The students were benefitting from the skills and guidance of these mentors. Other times, it is the students who assist and inspire our older players to re-learn their instrument and gain more confidence.

After the orchestra's first year, with both younger and older members reporting on its positive impact and modern approach, I thought, "Why shouldn't singers have the same opportunity?" The next year, the Eisner Intergenerational Choir was born. The Director of our Youth Music Programs suggested that, in addition to adding an intergenerational choir, we also create an intergenerational big band. This idea inspired me because of the extraordinary impact of connecting kids with musicians who grew up in the era of jazz. The year 2022 saw the birth of our choir and big band programs, bringing us to today with our three highly successful, lively, and ever-expanding Eisner Intergenerational Music Programs.

HOLA has over 120 active participants involved in the intergenerational orchestra, choir, and big band. We are excited to be a part of The Eisner Foundation's intergenerational portfolio and grateful for their generous support. During our season, which coincides with the academic year, rehearsals are offered weekly at our community center with performances often happening on campus and at other public venues. The multicultural and multigenerational music groups reflect the ethnicities and ages of community members who attend the concerts, strengthening the sense of community within our neighborhood.

Music is a wonderful, highly emotive, unifying and healing agent. Everyone contributes to the song, whether it's via their instrument or their voice. All ages, races, and genders can find a place to belong. In that moment, it's about humankind working toward a common goal of making something beautiful.

CARRIE BUCK

Former Executive Director, Homeless Intervention Services of Orange County (Founder of HomeShare OC)

his-oc.org

Matching aging homeowners with college students in need of affordable housing for mutual benefit.

"The more we work together and help each other, the more intrinsic benefits we receive from intergenerational partnerships."

When I was growing up in Indiana, my maternal grandmother lived several hours away. I only saw her a few times each year, and we were not particularly close, especially after the passing of my mother. But when I was in my early twenties, I needed a safe place to stay, and I showed up unannounced at my grandmother's doorstep. To my relief, she warmly welcomed me, saying, "Of course. Come in."

At the time, my grandmother was living alone and required surgery. The timing of my arrival proved fortuitous as I could assist her during her recovery. Neither of us ever imagined that we would be this close as adults. Through our shared living experience, an extraordinary bond developed between us, one that I did not have when I was little.

Later in my life, following my divorce, housing insecurity plagued me once again. With three children in tow and a nine-year work hiatus, I found myself on the brink of losing our home because I couldn't afford the house payments. The prospect of securing an apartment seemed equally unattainable, and moving in with my family was out of the question due to safety concerns. Additionally, I also wanted to finish my degree in Human Services, but the lack of resources posed a significant obstacle.

When my best friend said I could stay with her and her family, it saved me. Her parents took me in and didn't charge me rent. I stayed there for a year-and-a-half, got a job, and started saving money. Without them, I would likely have ended up homeless. Their generosity and faith in me changed my entire world and allowed me to get back on my feet. Later, they offered to loan me money for house payments and only charged me interest on the loan for a ten-year period. As a result, I ultimately finished school, became the executive director of a successful program, and began serving on the school board in my local community.

Their help made it possible for me to tackle some enormous challenges and fulfill some big dreams. These transformative experiences left a lasting impact on me, fostering a deep understanding and empathy towards individuals facing housing insecurity, grappling with adversity, and in need of essential support services.

In fact, my work at the Homeless Intervention Services of Orange County was centered on families and adults that needed assistance. Over time, I observed a rising number of service requests from older individuals and students. Startling statistics from the UCLA Center for the Transformation of Schools revealed that one in five community college students, one in ten California State University students, and one in twenty University of California students experienced homelessness within a year. These alarming figures underscore the urgent need for action and change.

When a grant centered on socially innovative programs became available, I remembered an intergenerational home-sharing story I'd heard of in Australia. It was fascinating, and I thought, "That's great. We don't have that in Orange County. We should do that." After some research, I wrote and submitted a co-housing proposal focused on our local colleges and senior community. We were awarded the grant, and that's how the HomeShare OC Program was created.

HomeShare OC matches housing-insecure college students with senior homeowners aged 55-plus who have an affordable room to rent. There are eligibility requirements and program guidelines. Students are often referred to us by colleges and universities, but sometimes find us on their own. Participating homeowners are usually discovered via presentations at senior centers or organizations like the Rotary or Kiwanis Clubs.

All participants complete a program application and questionnaire. These surveys help us find a good fit between students and older adults. We introduce them to one other via Zoom meetings, phone calls, and in person. If they decide to be roommates, we facilitate the completion of a shared living agreement. With that, we explore details and preferences that make up the dynamic of co-housing. Initially, they share a home for a semester, although this match may be extended once the initial period has been deemed a success and both parties agree.

Safety is also an important component of our program. Our participants go through background checks, and we inspect the houses to ensure that students have secure rooms, kitchen space to prepare nutritious meals, and a location that gives them safe access to school.

Monthly rent varies; however, it is capped at $500 so it's affordable for students working a part-time job. Without the pressure to work more hours, students have time to study, succeed in classes, and reach graduation. As part of their shared living agreement, students provide a minimum of five service hours per week, which may consist of household chores, companionship, or help with technology. Our staff is available to provide academic support and assist with any co-housing issues that arise.

The greatest challenge is finding enough homeowners. People are fearful. What I've found, however, is that when I take one of our homeowners along to a presentation, and the speaker talks about the benefits, it puts people at ease and helps them envision the possibilities. We have people sign up every time, and most of the homeowners that participate continue to receive new students each term.

The HomeShare OC Program, with its intergenerational component, serves several important roles. First, it addresses the housing crisis by providing dwelling spaces within the community's existing inventory. Second, it addresses social isolation by providing students and older adults with an opportunity to communicate and collaborate, despite different backgrounds, world viewpoints, and experience with technology. Third, it often transforms what was originally a financial need (by one or both parties) into an emotional bond or connection. And finally, as students take responsibility for their own lives during this pivotal period, many move forward from junior college to a four-year university, graduate with their degree, or apply to graduate school.

As I know from personal experience, just one person saying, "I can help you," has the potential to create a profound impact. The home-sharing program is just one strategy that we used to combat homelessness, social disconnection, and loneliness in our community. The trust that develops between students and older homeowners results in discovering similarities, sharing stories, giving and receiving advice, teaching life lessons, and experiencing mentoring that goes both directions. The more we work together and help each other, the more the intrinsic benefits we receive from intergenerational partnerships.

DONNA BUTTS

Executive Director, Generations United

gu.org

Improving the lives of children, youth, and older people through intergenerational collaboration, public policies, and programs for the enduring benefit of all.

"We believe in a world that values and engages all generations."

I came to this work because I love teenagers. Until I heard about Generations United, I had devoted my life to working with teens, just as the adults in my life had been dedicated to seeing me reach adulthood despite myself.

As the teen director at the Salem, Oregon, YWCA, I ran a program called Senior Outreach. It matched high school sociology students with low-income older adults living on their own in senior housing. After a semester of weekly visits, many of them became close. The end of the session potluck dinner was quite an affair, with both generations dressed in their finest. There were tears but more often no long goodbyes, just plans to see each other again soon. They had become friends, drawn together by purpose. They thought they were going to be helping the other; they ended up helping themselves.

There were kids who skipped school except for the day they were supposed to visit the older adult they were matched with. There were seniors who didn't get out of bed in the morning and open the curtains except for the day their student was scheduled to visit. They both had purpose, a reason to show up.

They saw each other across the age gap and found acceptance. Such was the case with an unlikely pairing. The photograph of them in the local paper said it all. She was in her eighties with silver hair, and she's reaching across the table to pat his hand. He's sixteen, in a black leather jacket with an orange mohawk haircut. The caption read, "He may look a little strange, but he's such a nice boy."

When Generations United was newly incorporated and looking for an executive director, I remembered those unlikely friends, and thought more older adults should be in the lives of teens. They were growing in numbers and had time. Plus, I could help create the world I wanted to grow old in. So, I said 'yes' and became Generations United's executive director in 1997. I never looked back.

As the champion for intergenerational solutions for more than thirty-five years, Generations United focuses on programs and policies that connect generations and value people at all ages and stages of life. Our goal is to be the bridge that brings together groups that traditionally focus on specific age demographics. We push for a unified agenda and ensure our distinctive voice is heard during public debates.

We deeply believe that intergenerational collaboration strengthens our communities, boosts our economy, and is the foundation for crafting public policies that cater to the needs of every generation. For us, it's crucial to use resources in ways that connect generations rather than separate them. Furthermore, promoting diversity, equity, and inclusion in all our intergenerational initiatives is a cornerstone of our mission. We emphasize the importance of involving people with varied real-life experiences in every aspect of our work. Last, we can't help but honor the grandparents and other adults who step up to raise children. We see their immense contribution not only as a familial bond but also as an invaluable economic service to our nation.

Intergenerational programs are based on reciprocity and respect, breaking down artificial age barriers by connecting, often deeply, two or more generations. As our country's population evolves, people are waking up to smell the demographics and increasingly realizing connecting different age groups is essential, although not always easy.

People are aging and experiencing their longer lives differently than previous generations. While some are content to withdraw from society, many more are hungry to remain engaged and live with purpose rather than feel irrelevant. They see potential. With regular interaction with younger age groups, older adults report feeling more connected, take better care of themselves, score higher on memory tests and feel more optimistic.

For younger age groups, they learn soft skills that range from patience to tolerance. They gain comfort and coping skills from people who have lived through joyful and tough times, as well as a sense of roots and connection. They too feel purpose and are less likely to fear their own aging.

Intergenerational programs embrace diversity, squelch ageism, and inspire hope. At a time when so much attention is focused on what divides us, these programs bring out what is best in our neighborhoods and communities: compassion, cooperation and acceptance across a myriad of divides. At Generations United, we are the convener, educator, elevator, and standard setter for high quality intergenerational practices providing tools and platforms that strengthen this critical work nationwide. We are honored to do this work because we profoundly believe we are stronger together.

ALISON CLYDE

Generations Working Together

generationsworkingtogether.org

Generations Working Together is the nationally recognized center of excellence supporting the development and integration of intergenerational work across Scotland.

"The true value of intergenerational connections lies in the profound impact they have on individuals and society."

My personal journey into intergenerational work began during my tenure at a local charity that initially focused on a randomized medical control study related to cardiology. This study explored the concept of mentoring for individuals who had experienced coronary issues. Over the course of ten years, I became involved in the study's expansion into the community, where we aimed to test whether the successful medical study could be applied in a broader context.

It was during this time that I encountered various individuals and organizations, each with their own unique focus and scope in the field of intergenerational work. I was also aware of various articles published by the Beth Johnson Foundation, which enriched my understanding of how connecting generations could benefit individuals with coronary heart disease, given the social and emotional aspects of their condition. This idea started to take root in my mind, even though I was not actively seeking a job in this field at the time.

An unexpected opportunity arose when I noticed a National Coordinator position for Scotland aiming to establish a National Center for Intergenerational Practice. I decided to pursue this role and have now dedicated twelve years to Generations Working Together (GWT). Established in 2007, GWT officially became a charity in 2015 and has played a pivotal role in Scotland's intergenerational landscape.

At GWT, our mission is to support and promote intergenerational work throughout Scotland. In 2020 we launched our call for Scotland to become the first intergenerational nation. We provide resources, knowledge, and networking opportunities for individuals and organizations across various sectors. Our primary goal is to facilitate meaningful connections between younger and older generations, ensuring that these initiatives are well-planned and executed effectively.

Due to the pandemic, we encountered a multitude of challenges, one of which put an abrupt halt to our efforts. However, amid these challenges, a significant shift occurred in how we perceived our purpose. It transitioned from being considered a mere 'nice thing to do' to something utterly essential. It became evident that those who recognized its essential nature were the ones truly dedicated to making a difference. Our traditional perspective on connecting older adults and young people revolved around scenarios like seniors from care homes briefly engaging with young people to share their World War II experiences with students. These encounters, often fleeting, no longer sufficed. We aimed to flip this narrative and emphasize the importance of lasting impact and longevity in our approach.

To bring this vision to life, we initiated a funding application with the UK's National Lottery. Collaborating with organizations such as Linked Generations Northern Ireland, Apples and Honey Nightingale, and the Welsh Intergenerational Network, along with our own organization, Generations Working Together, we embarked on a mission to develop a toolkit to support our efforts. This toolkit was designed to be tested by thirty diverse projects, spanning various age groups, from early years to young adults, and covering a wide array of themes.

Our objective was to empower both newcomers and seasoned practitioners alike by providing them with a toolkit that could enhance their practices and improve the quality of their projects. Central to this approach was the idea of fostering better relationships and partnerships within these projects. Instead of relying on a single individual within an organization to understand and implement these goals, our aim was for two individuals from different organizations to undergo training and gain a comprehensive understanding of the concept. This way, if one person faced challenges like illness or a job change, the connection could remain intact, ensuring the project's continuity.

Our efforts weren't limited to project participants and organizers; we also recognized the positive effect on staff members. Engaging in intergenerational connections was found to be highly rewarding for them. Additionally, we sought to address the concerns some families had about our practices, particularly those involving end-of-life scenarios. It was crucial to highlight the incredible importance of these interactions. The Quality Indicators Toolkit, developed over two and a half years, emerged as the cornerstone of our endeavor. Rooted in four key domains—levels of engagement and the principles of intergenerational work—it was informed by rigorous academic research conducted in collaboration with esteemed institutions worldwide.

We emphasized the importance of quantifying the social value created by purposefully connecting generations through a social return on investment analysis, recognizing that securing funding and support hinged on such evaluations. Our aspiration is for the Quality Indicators Toolkit to be widely acknowledged as the gold standard for quality intergenerational work in the UK. Projects adhering to its principles and effectively using the toolkit could earn accreditation, signifying their commitment to this social initiative.

Ultimately, our goal is to ensure that intergenerational work is not merely a fleeting trend but a sustainable, impactful practice. It's about building communities, reducing ageism, and addressing social isolation and loneliness through meaningful relationships. The distinction between multigenerational and intergenerational is of utmost importance. These two concepts are fundamentally different, and it is crucial to understand their unique characteristics and objectives. Multigenerational settings often involve diverse age groups coexisting within a shared space, such as a large building or facility. However, the key differentiator lies in the nature of their interactions. In multigenerational environments, individuals from different age groups may merely pass by one another without engaging in meaningful activities or connections. It's akin to parallel existence, where age groups coexist but do not collaborate or share experiences. Conversely, an intergenerational community fosters a deep sense of connection and collaboration among individuals of varying age groups.

Picture a community center where a youth group actively interacts with older individuals, participating in joint activities, sharing stories, and building relationships. In such settings, people not only know one another but also engage in genuine conversations, be it at a cafe or during shared events. These interactions result in the development of meaningful relationships that transcend age boundaries.

The essence of intergenerational work goes beyond providing a service; it is centered on building enduring connections among generations. Unfortunately, some individuals may misconstrue this initiative as mere interactions or connections, failing to grasp its true depth and significance. Thus, there is an imperative need for greater understanding of the concept's true essence. Intergenerational work is not a fleeting trend; rather, it should be a long-term commitment to building and nurturing relationships across generations. Its long-term effect extends far beyond immediate outcomes, as it serves as a catalyst for social change, particularly in reducing ageism and addressing issues of social isolation and loneliness.

In 2021, we launched Global Intergenerational Week, which serves as an annual celebration dedicated to all aspects of intergenerational engagement. Bringing together fifteen countries from around the world to celebrate all things intergenerational, this campaign aims to ignite inspiration within individuals, groups, organizations, as well as local and national governments, and non-governmental organizations (NGOs) to wholeheartedly embrace intergenerational practices. These practices involve intentionally connecting people from various generations through activities that mutually benefit all participants.

The week provides a unique opportunity to acknowledge and applaud exemplary practices, innovative ideas, meaningful moments, and local initiatives that bring together different age groups, fostering the creation of friendships between people who might not ordinarily meet. It encourages the global community to come together and exchange insights, showcasing creative and effective methods of bridging generational gaps on a worldwide platform.

The true value of intergenerational connections lies in the profound impact they have on individuals and society. Through my twelve years at GWT, I have witnessed the transformative power of these interactions. These connections have the potential to reshape our societal fabric and enhance our collective well-being. It's not merely about the activities themselves; it's about people from different generations getting to know each other on a deeper level. GWT serves as a catalyst for positive change, providing the resources, knowledge, and support needed to bridge generational divides and build stronger, more connected communities.

RACHEL B. COHEN, MSW, MUP

Executive Director, LinkAGES

linkAGESconnects.org

Preventing and reducing loneliness and social isolation among youth and older adults through high-quality intergenerational programs designed to connect generations, decrease ageism, and support healthier communities.

"Looking at the world around me, I see multi-colored threads woven together into tapestries of community. Communities—whether rooted in geography, culture, or identity—exist where people feel a deep sense of belonging to one another and the land."

I am a bridge builder and an interpreter within, and between, communities. I facilitate collaboration across sectors, lending my expertise in social services, housing, community development, environmental education, aging, and food systems. For more than twenty-five years, I have helped entities understand and work with one another to achieve common goals on the local, statewide, and national level. By leveraging funds, staff, knowledge, and networks, my clients and I work together to build communities that are supportive, engaging, and equitable places to grow up and grow older.

In 2016, I founded Aging Dynamics, a national consulting practice with a commitment to integrity, trust, curiosity, and inclusion. Our clients are purpose-driven organizations, building communities that are healthy places to grow up and grow older. Aging Dynamics' services include strategic planning, capacity building and technical assistance, facilitation, building collaboratives and coalitions, and designing and executing inclusive community engagement efforts. Our clients include the Denver Art Museum, Volunteers of America, foundations, cities, counties, and more.

Aging Dynamics' mission and work is exemplified in our project LinkAGES, a multi-sector collaborative launched in 2018. LinkAGES addresses social isolation and loneliness across ages by creating meaningful opportunities for intergenerational connections. Aging Dynamics acts as the backbone organization to LinkAGES, providing a suite of services that includes program design, partnership matchmaking, marketing, and more. Member organizations collaborate with one another and community partners to offer high-quality intergenerational programs, demonstrably reducing loneliness in youth, social isolation in older adults and ageism in both. Aging Dynamics works to remove any barrier that prevents them from doing so.

We constantly evaluate and adapt both LinkAGES programs and the collaborative itself to have greater impact both collectively and individually. This supported backbone model has been successful in significantly increasing the number of quality intergenerational programs, reducing feelings of isolation, increasing confidence of members to partner and develop new programs.

There is so much value in intergeneration programs, and I've seen many positive outcomes.

The memories of my childhood, adolescence, and early adulthood are filled with the loving, steadfast presence of my uncle. Then, abruptly, those memories cease. My uncle was unmarried and child-free, geographically separated from his family and network. He slipped into social isolation and loneliness that permeated his home and heart. He died alone, and the world was robbed too soon of a kind, generous, social justice warrior. It did not have to be this way.

Intergenerational programs connect us to community and help us feel purpose and belonging. This is something so many people lack in a world where families scatter across the country, retirement cuts off lifelong social networks, and kids are experiencing unprecedented levels of loneliness.

When people don't feel connected to others, they can experience social isolation (a lack of social connections) or loneliness (a subjective feeling like hunger). We measure social isolation and loneliness as unique experiences. Both, however, can decrease our quality of life and hurt our physical and mental health—at every age.

Research has directly linked social isolation in older adults with higher rates of depression, anxiety, substance abuse, heart disease, stroke, and shorter life spans. At the 2017 Annual Convention of the American Psychological Association, psychologist Julianne Hold-Lunstad said, "There is robust evidence that social isolation and loneliness significantly increase risk for premature mortality, and the magnitude of the risk exceeds that of many leading health indicators."

Meaningful intergenerational connections are about *mutuality*. Everyone involved is seen and valued for who they are and what they contribute. The best programs are designed around a shared activity and treat all participants like equals. Whether it's creating art, making music, or giving back (together), at the heart is human connection.

Connecting across generations is linked to positive physical and mental health outcomes. Youth can experience heightened empathy, increased confidence and self-esteem, and decreased loneliness. Older adults report reduced symptoms of depression, enhanced sense of purpose, and decreased experience of social isolation.

Psychologist Abraham Maslow put love and belonging at the center of his Hierarchy of Needs, aware of the fact that a sense of deeper connection is what gives life meaning. In her book, *Belong*, Radha Argawal reimagined the Hierarchy of Needs and placed belonging at the very foundation of the hierarchy, as significant as food, water, and shelter. She even put love and positive touch here. Argawal defines belonging as a feeling of deep relatedness and acceptance.

Around the world, community-based organizations, senior housing facilities, businesses, and governments have been exploring how to alleviate the social isolation and loneliness that disproportionately impact older adults, adolescents, and young people 18-25 years old. What have they found? Connecting these age groups with one another in meaningful ways is one key part of the puzzle.

So why aren't intergenerational programs more readily available in communities around the world?

Significant barriers to intergenerational programming are most often rooted in a lack of money, time, and staff. They include:

- **Funding:** Most available charitable funding is highly restricted to specific outcomes and age groups, and this rarely includes intergenerational programs.
- **Evaluation:** Without proof that a program elicits results, it's challenging to find more funding to run it again. It's also difficult to know what's working and what needs to be improved to sustain it.

- **Collaboration:** Intergenerational programs require two or more organizations to collaborate. Identifying and building trusting relationships is complex and time-intensive, and often there simply isn't money earmarked for this type of work in organizational budgets.
- **Program Design:** Designing a meaningful program that both older adults and youth want to participate in requires special knowledge, tools, and commitment.

Intergenerational programs, when designed well, benefit individuals, organizations, and communities. Their impact ripples across entire human systems, like families, schools, and towns. Participants of LinkAGES will ask to become involved in more programs, and some even participate in the same program again in order to meet new people and create new connections. Other participants maintain the connections they made through a program, and begin to build a broader network. For instance, an older couple who took part in a photography program, where they were matched with an undergraduate student, continued to meet regularly for dinner, even after the program ended. They also invited other students to join, broadening and deepening the connections made during the program. These connections beget more connections as people get more comfortable and confident with sharing experiences with people of different ages. A successful intergenerational program creates meaningful connections between ages. A meaningful connection is when two people come to a mutual recognition that, despite the decades of age between them, they share so much in common. A profound connection can occur in the space of weeks, years, or a lifetime—and they all alter the trajectory of our lives and how we see ourselves.

CHIP CONLEY

Co-Founder and CEO, MEA (Modern Elder Academy)

meawisdom.com

Dedicated to reframing the concept of aging.

"We are the first ever 'midlife wisdom school' dedicated to guiding and supporting adults through periods of transition in life."

I think I've always been fascinated by the concept of intergenerational connections. It all started with my grandmother, Nani, that I deeply admired and wanted to be like. She was just happy all the time and always had a big smile on her face. She had a strong point of view, but she also had a lot of compassion.

But it wasn't until I was 52 years old and I joined Airbnb that I realized the power of intergenerational collaboration in the workplace. At the time, this tiny little tech startup wanted to democratize hospitality. I was working very closely with the three founders who were all two decades younger than me, the average age there was 26. I loved the 'generational potluck' we created. I could bring to the table some of my lived experience and wisdom, which I define as metabolized experience that leads to distilled compassion. They could bring their knowledge and wisdom, as well as their fresh perspectives. I started calling myself a 'mentern', a mentor and an intern at the same time. I believe that we live in an era where the best way for organizations to help foster learning and development is through mutual mentorship across generations.

In my role at Airbnb, I noticed the distinct qualities of young and older brains. As a generalization, a young brain tends to be fast and focused, and has great fluid intelligence, and is very logical and able to solve problems adeptly. Older brains, while shrinking physically, develop what I like to call a 'four-wheel drive of the brain.' What starts to become more prominent is crystallized intelligence. Crystallized intelligence is different than fluid intelligence in that it is not about being fast and focused, it's about being holistic and systemic, and being strong. It's being good at connecting the dots.

If you put together a room of people who have fluid intelligence and crystallized intelligence and various life experiences, you can create a synergistic relationship, where the best of both worlds creates an even better world. I experienced that at Airbnb in so many ways. I'm proud to say that I think the company is a better place because one of the things I tried to do is say, "Hey, we can't just all be millennials here. We need some Gen Xers. We need some boomers. We need to take age diversity as seriously as we take gender, race, and sexual orientation diversity." And we were one of the first companies in Silicon Valley that advocated for age diversity, stressing its importance alongside other forms of diversity.

After Airbnb, I created MEA (Modern Elder Academy), partly because I had two experiences of midlife, one terrible one, one great. The terrible experience was between ages 45 and 49, where everything that could go wrong *did* go wrong. Other than getting a midlife crisis book or talking to my best friend, who was a coach, I didn't really have a lot of resources, and I sort of felt like I was getting the game of life wrong. This was also the time of the great recession, and during that time I lost five friends, all men, aged 42-52 to suicide. And so, note to self, *this midlife thing is challenging.*

Then I went into my fifties and made a bunch of changes in my life, a lot of transition, and I had the best decade of my life. The proof of happiness research shows that as we get older, after about age 50 on average (your mileage may vary), we see a growing contentment in our life. I saw my fifties as being like, *wow, I'm solidly in midlife and I'm loving it.*

What I wanted to do by creating MEA was to establish the world's first midlife wisdom school, a place where we really looked at how do we cultivate and harvest wisdom because people rarely recognize they even have it. And then, how do we make a difference in the world with that wisdom? But most important, how do we help people realize that midlife is not a crisis, but it's a chrysalis? And a chrysalis means it is the dark, gooey, solitary time when transformation happens. If you're going to go through a dark, gooey, solitary time, why not do it with a bunch of other people who are going through that time and are helping to foster each other's transformation? That's why I created MEA.

I think midlife is sort of like middle age. There are no boundaries for it. And sometimes people think that they're in midlife at age 30, and sometimes they think they're in midlife at age 80. It's sort of hard to say, especially in a world where more and more people are living to 100.

It's called the Modern Elder Academy because that's what they called me at Airbnb. And they said, "A modern elder is someone who is as curious as they are wise." I didn't expect to get millennials applying to come to a place with 'elder' in the title, but what I came to realize that over 15% of our people who come are millennials. In any workshop, we have at least three generations in the room together. Our average age of people who come to MEA is 54, but in any workshop, you might have people as young as 28 and as old as 88. It's very cross-generational.

We also have specific workshops on intergenerational wisdom. The full intent of those is to help people learn from each other across the generations, and to look at how do we develop that. I think it's an essential part of a pluralistic society. One of our workshop leaders, Mark Friedman from CoGenerate (formerly Encore.org) said, "The issue we have in the world today is no longer, 'how do we help take people into their second act to do something for good for the world?' No, our big issue is 'how do we create a new generational compact?'"

What's fascinating is how MEA has evolved to include participants across a wide age spectrum. This diversity enriches the learning experience and reflects the fluidity of what we consider 'midlife.' In a world where life expectancy is increasing, the boundaries of midlife are expanding, making this phase of life an ongoing journey of discovery for many, regardless of their age.

SUE EGERSDORFF

Founder, Ready Generations

readygenerations.co.uk

Making a difference to lifelong learning and care by becoming a leading provider of intergenerational practice and provision.

"Connecting generations has the ability to foster reciprocity, empathy, and citizenship while instilling respect and dignity as inherent human rights, irrespective of age."

My journey into the world of intergenerational work began in a rather unexpected manner, having been rooted in my lifelong career as an early year's educator. For four decades, I dedicated myself to fostering early childhood development and, in the process, contributed to national policies in the UK's educational landscape. However, my transition into intergenerational work was not premeditated, rather, it was catalyzed by a deeply personal experience.

As I ventured closer to retirement, my life took an unexpected turn when my mother's health began to deteriorate rapidly. Until that point, I had never truly encountered the realm of adult social care. It was during this challenging period that I watched my mother's world, once vibrant and expansive, shrink before my eyes. The stark contrast between her former life and her growing isolation left an indelible mark on me. Witnessing her frustration and disenfranchisement as a brilliant woman suddenly unable to engage with the world due to health issues, was profoundly unsettling. The experience compelled me to confront the reality of older people's care, the marginalization they often endure, and their pervasive isolation. Although my mother is no longer with us, her memory fuels my determination to reshape the narrative around living well in older age and continuing to find purpose and meaning in life.

It was at this juncture that a remarkable opportunity emerged—a chance to redefine the way society perceives and provides care for both young children and older people. A care provider called Belong Villages in the northwest of England approached me with a unique proposal. They were in the process of constructing a progressive care village concept that incorporated independent living, residential care, nursing and end-of-life care, all within a single, comprehensive complex. In this grand vision, there was an underutilized space in the building, and the idea was born to integrate a nursery within this environment. Given my expertise in early childhood development and education, they sought my advice on establishing this nursery.

However, I found myself at a crossroads. I was unwilling to propose a conventional commissioning model, whereby a nursery provider was brought in without deeper considerations of the potential of the model. Instead, I proposed a bold alternative: let us reimagine the entire framework of care for both young families and older people. I advocated for a fully integrated living model, one that transcended the boundaries of co-location. It wasn't about having a nursery adjacent to a care home; it was about creating an ecosystem where generations lived side by side, as in the vibrant neighborhoods I recalled from my own upbringing.

This visionary approach necessitated navigating challenging conversations, overcoming some resistance and being prepared to work with integrity as partners in a new venture. Belong Villages were brave partners, agreeing to adopt my unconventional perspective on the project. We began to explore and consider its potential to change lives in a sustained way over time through relational approaches that placed people at the forefront of decision making. It was at this juncture that I realized my retirement plans had taken an unexpected turn. To ensure the enduring legacy of this project, I established a charity called Ready Generations, with an amazing colleague, Liz Ludden, who already ran an outstanding nursery in Liverpool. Together, we made it clear from the outset that our goal was not financial reward but to inspire future generations and provoke change within the existing care infrastructure through practical, evidence-based research.

What we have cultivated over the past sixteen months transcends the boundaries of a typical nursery or care home. It is an innovation-seeking research model with affiliations to eight UK universities. Our nursery is not only a childcare facility; it is a living laboratory where we are constantly asking questions and observing what works for people and what helps them to succeed and enjoy life whatever their circumstance. The outcomes have surpassed all my hopes, and we are now able to make a genuinely authentic contribution to professional forums and academic papers that are beginning to garner increased interest and recognition. This was precisely what I envisioned for the latter part of my career—to write, challenge, and hopefully inspire those who follow, encouraging them to embrace and further this transformative concept.

Our journey has yielded a rich array of findings, some encouraging, others profoundly thought-provoking. What has struck me most is that age is no barrier to the basic human need for dignity, connection and a sense of belonging. We are always better together than alone. Whether one is 8 months old or 98 years old, the fundamental aspects of attachment, empathy, contribution, and meaningful relationships remain the same. This insight led us to develop our bespoke Mirrored Curriculum Framework (MCF), a blueprint for lifelong learning that blurs age distinctions and fosters an environment where all individuals, regardless of age, are effective and progressive learners and educators in equal measure.

In our inclusive and collaborative community, we have witnessed a transformation in the way generations relate to one another. Instead of demarcating roles, we have embraced a model where older people are encouraged to lead learning by using their knowledge, experience, and wisdom to actively assume the role of educator. This shift has been significant in how older people see themselves and their importance, instilling a sense of continued purpose and responsibility for others that is powerful and motivating. For many, this shift has elevated their stature from passive care recipients to active contributors. The results have been profound—our staff-to-child ratio has essentially become a ratio of 50 potential educators to 25 children. This provides just what young learners need, interested adults with time to spend listening, observing and extending learning opportunities and experiences.

The impact on the children is remarkable. Vocabulary, word knowledge, sentence structure, problem solving, and social-emotional skills have all progressed rapidly. We're now focusing on developing more academically robust measures to substantiate these qualitative observations. Beyond cognitive development, children are learning critical life skills such as reciprocity, empathy, compassion and tenderness, all essential elements of personal agency, identity and citizenship central to knowing oneself and participating in the building of stable and compassionate societies.

Our approach reaches beyond education. It aims to re-orientate care and education systems toward greater equity and social justice. It prioritizes attention to the detail of how people experience life, particularly at the margins. This intimate noticing increasingly involves scrutiny of even seemingly minor aspects of life, like paying attention to how food is served, room décor, and lighting and noise pollution. We've paid attention to often overlooked aspects of daily living alongside recognizing the significance of small things and acts to people. This focus on noticing the detail of people's lives and developing a set of operating principles that place equity and inclusion as central is impacting on confidence, autonomy and self-agency, helping the most vulnerable to feel that modern life is less precarious for them. To support autonomy and risk taking throughout the life course, we are also developing creative ways of thinking about active living at every age. This includes exploring new ideas about healthy motor development, balance, posture and co-ordination.

What makes this endeavor truly exciting for me is its unpredictability and challenge to the accepted status quo. Our journey is taking us down unexpected paths, as we let children and older people lead us into understanding of what matters most to them, makes them feel safe and allows them to be who they are meant to be. We are embracing indigenous knowledge from all over the world, which provides a wealth of wisdom about identity, culture and multigenerational living. The wonderfully rich nature of our discoveries is testament to the boundless potential of intergenerational interactions and the aspirational connectivity they bring.

As I reflect on this journey, I see it as a profound opportunity to make what has become invisible, visible again. In many ways, it is a journey of return to some lost ways of living together that recognize individual roles and accountabilities and yet garner a sense of togetherness and responsibility for others. This is powerful for older people, providing a renewed sense of purpose and identity, whilst for children, imparts a broader sense of agency, community and citizenship. It's all about fostering the competencies that bring people together to find solutions collaboratively. Just caring is not enough at this moment in time. We need to care more about ourselves and each other. I believe professional educators and carers are incredible people who want to work in a system that respects social justice and leads to more interaction and connection between learners of all ages. Currently, the siloed way of providing services by segregating and separating is only increasing isolation and loss of hope. Instilling respect and dignity as inherent human rights, irrespective of age, presents a compelling rationale for change.

As we move forward, our vision is extending beyond the definition of intergenerational work. We are thinking more and more about what it means to be part of a community, a neighborhood, a street. It feels like some of the boundaried arrangements we accept in education and care need to be dismantled to allow new ideas to flourish rather than layering new ideas onto systems that are buckling under pressure and which are, all too often, reactive rather than preventative in scope. Whatever the future brings, we will remain committed to working with heart, listening and hearing the quietest of voices. We will not rush and will work at a pace that includes everyone, not shying away from the complexities inherent in many stubborn, hard-to-shift issues. Making systems stutter and slow down is an innovative way to allow new leaders to emerge with a cohesive view of how to shape a more compassionate, inclusive, and joyful society.

ANNEKE FITZGERALD, PH.D.

Emeritus Professor, Australian Institute for Intergenerational Practice

aiip.net.au

Re-connecting communities through the development, implementation and evaluation of intergenerational programs.

"Our long-term vision is for intergenerational interactions and programs to be a normal part of our everyday life in both formal and informal settings."

In 2013, my daughter Kimberley and I had a cup of tea and a chat about our workday around the kitchen table. My daughter, who was an early learning educator at the time, was telling me about her trials and tribulations around tasks associated with caring for children. As a former registered nurse of 20-plus years who has worked in Aged Care, I sympathized with her and shared some of my stories around caring for older people. In chatting, we discovered and concluded that caring for younger and older people isn't so different. My daughter asked, “If it is so similar, why is it not combined more?” This question was the start of our intergenerational practice journey.

We quickly established a small team to explore what is known about combining care for older people and younger people. We learned that childcare falls under education and aged care falls under health. We decided that, for regulatory reasons, intergenerational care should probably fall under education. We then established the importance of health economics, business planning, and career development for sustained intergenerational practice. And we attracted other disciplines into our group, especially those with experience in early learning and childcare.

We learned that many organizations are involved in an intergenerational practice of sorts; however, we also discovered that intergenerational practice is seldom planned, organized, and evaluated. Additionally, there is little to no evidence base for best intergenerational practices. This became the foundation to our work today, eight years later: a sustainable curriculum base with planned and evaluated programs bringing people together for a specific purpose.

While the intergenerational team was establishing the research for best practices in different modes of intergenerational practices (Dementia and Aged Services Fund 2017-1019), and establishing alternative programs such as intergenerational learning via videoconferencing, we also started to look to the future. We developed our mission and vision and distributed our toolkit. In doing so, we expanded our network far and wide, nationally and internationally.

Over time, the Intergenerational Care Program became the Intergenerational Learning Program, which evolved into intergenerational practices to ensure inclusiveness of all forms of intergenerational care, learning, and practices. Now we are on the cusp of our next adventure: The Australian Institute for Intergenerational Practice. We want to bring people together to ensure the best intergenerational experiences possible and to normalize intergenerational connections in Australia.

To view an ever-growing collection of organizations conducting intergenerational research or practice around Australia, visit: https://bit.ly/4aVPqBT

TRACEY GENDRON, MS, PH.D.

Author of Ageism Unmasked
Chair and Professor, Department of Gerontology
Virginia Commonwealth University
Executive Director, Virginia Center on Aging

gerontology.chp.vcu.edu

Executive Director, Virginia Center on Aging

vcoa.chp.vcu.edu

Ageism Unmasked is peeling back the layers to expose how cultural norms and unconscious prejudices have seeped into our lives, silently shaping our treatment of others based on their age and our own misconceptions about aging—and about ourselves.

"We need to let go of our desperate need to stay young, and understand how we personally, systematically, structurally, and institutionally stigmatize being old."

I have always enjoyed spending time with elders. However, my true passion for intergenerational relationships began with my grandparents. I grew up spending time with Nonny and Poppy almost every week. We spent Sundays at their house watching football, listening to classical music, baking and eating four-course meals that Nonny prepared herself. They came to all of my recitals, school events and participated in special occasions. My brother and I stayed with them when my parents traveled, and I have fond memories of Poppy's fractured fairy tales (stories reminiscent of fairy tales but with his unique version of humor) and Nonny popping popcorn on the stove without the lid on the pot (by accident, but we had wonderful laughs). I learned so much from them, but I also felt that they learned from me. They took a genuine interest in the things that I did and the experiences that I had. I couldn't have predicted at the time that this organic relationship would have such a profound impact on my life, but it did.

I took that love of being with my grandparents to my academic studies. When I learned of the word 'gerontology', I knew that this was the career that I wanted to pursue. Through gerontology, I learned that younger and older people spending time together was the most effective way to ensure positive attitudes about aging. I realized how privileged I was that I had the opportunity for organic intergenerational learning as I grew up. Until recently, I didn't think about this as 'intergenerational work' because it just felt natural and normal to be a part of my life. I also learned that many others are not afforded the same early positive experiences that I was, and instead, realized that they learned about aging and older people through mass media and negative cultural messages portraying old as a feared and dreaded state of being.

I am now driven to think about intergenerational work intentionally, and I support the work of so many others who strive to provide opportunities for intergenerational engagement. I also maintain an intentional practice in my own life to surround myself with an age-diverse mix of people. This diversity of experience and perspective enriches me in countless ways. Learning from others' lived experiences enriches my understanding of the world and provides me with the tools to navigate it better.

Intergenerational living provided ample opportunities for children, adults and elders to live, work and grow together. Living in intergenerational households was the norm in the United States as late as the 19th century. The Industrial Revolution changed the landscape, and people moved away from family farms into cities where jobs were located. This resulted in a drastic change to the structure of family systems, and intergenerational households slowly dissipated. One side effect of the decreased organic relationships between younger and older people was the amplification of negative attitudes about aging.

We now use intergenerational programs to help create purposeful opportunities for people of different ages to interact and learn from each other. Robust literature describes the benefits of intergenerational engagement for younger and older people (Carr, 2016), including the benefit of improving attitudes about aging and decreasing ageism (Burnes et al., 2019).

However, intergenerational programming must go beyond the stereotypical version of younger people 'serving' older people to be the most beneficial. The key to effective intergenerational programs is to create reciprocal learning where both older and younger people benefit. My colleagues and I developed one such program that brings together students in the health professions with older adults in the community to provide them with the opportunity for purposeful conversation. This program aims to have older adults share their experiences growing older and navigating healthcare services with students in healthcare fields. Students ask their older adult mentors guiding questions such as, "What is a difficult experience you have had with a healthcare provider?" And, "What advice do you have for me as a healthcare practitioner?" Both students and older adult mentors have reported tremendous growth and learning from engaging in this type of dialogue together.

Intergenerational relationships provide opportunities for perspective building and are one of the most effective tools to improve attitudes about aging and older people. When we spend time with people of different ages, we learn that we share more commonalities with people than we ever could have realized.

Sources:

Burnes, D., Sheppard, C., Henderson Jr, C. R., Wassel, M., Cope, R., Barber, C., & Pillemer, K. (2019). Interventions to reduce ageism against older adults: A systematic review and meta-analysis. *American Journal of Public Health,* 109(8), e1-e9.

Carr, D. C., & Gunderson, J. A. (2016). The third age of life: Leveraging the mutual benefits of intergenerational engagement. *Public Policy & Aging Report,* 26(3), 83-87.

MARIA GENNÉ

Founder and Director, Kairos Alive!

kairosalive.org

Building our community and enabling people of all ages and abilities to experience the joy of movement.

"We are transforming lives through dance and story, raising awareness of the importance of creative involvement across the lifespan, as people from diverse backgrounds and ages come together, move, and connect through the universal language of dance."

Dancing has always been a part of who I am, almost like a language of its own. Growing up, I had a unique family background that shaped my interest in intergenerational connections. After my father's untimely passing, my family moved to live close to my aunt, his sister, which brought me into close contact with various aunts, uncles, and my mother's remarkable history. My mother, an influential figure in my life, had a significant impact on my perspective. As a young woman, she served as the first field secretary for the National NAACP, working alongside prominent figures like Roy Wilkins and Thurgood Marshall. She traveled across the northern United States, advocating for intercultural education, a concept that fascinated me.

Dance and music have always been my preferred modes of expression, my true languages. Early on, I started nurturing this passion by taking care of neighborhood kids and introducing them to the joy of dancing. At 16, my dance teacher suggested that I take over children's dance classes, an opportunity that allowed me to develop my own creative approach to dance education, emphasizing exploration, discovery, and creativity over rigid steps and aesthetics.

Through my college years in North Dakota, I immersed myself at The Center for Teaching and Learning, which embraced progressive education and intergenerational community building. This experience expanded my understanding of the power of different-age learning and inspired me to create my graduate program, teaching creative dance and creative dramatics to future elementary, high school, and early childhood teachers.

My professional career began with a job at a dance company in Fargo, ND/Moorhead, MN, where I was responsible for the children's program, as well as performing. I realized that my true passion lay in fostering creative connections across generations and backgrounds. When I moved to Minneapolis and started my family, I taught creative dance classes and eventually established family dance classes to cater to my new role as a parent.

In 1987, I founded Young Dance, a dance company focused on working with children and teenagers. I enfranchised children to be full creative contributors in an intergenerational environment. This venture allowed me to continue my pursuit of creating together across generational boundaries. I observed the transformative power of dance and music in bridging these gaps, whether it was young children dancing with high school students or families dancing together.

My involvement with schools, both as a specialist and as a classroom teacher, revealed to me the incredible potential of dance and music in fostering whole-brain learning and allowing students to discover their creative capacities. It was heartening to witness children and adults alike experiencing the joy of dance, gaining confidence, and achieving success through this form of expression.

As I continued my journey, I felt the need to create something more profound—a platform that would bring people of different ages, abilities, and cultural backgrounds together through dance, music, and storytelling. In 1999, the idea for an intergenerational dance company was born, which eventually became Kairos Dance Theatre (now Kairos Alive!). The name 'Kairos' signifies the open moment in time, capturing the essence of the experiences we aim to create.

Kairos Alive! focuses on creating intergenerational dance halls where professional artists, community members, elders, and children come together to dance and celebrate life. These events are carefully curated to accommodate individuals with varying mobility, ensuring everyone can participate and enjoy the transformative power of dance.

Over the years, our work has evolved to encompass a broader range of intergenerational and intercultural programs. We have adapted to the digital age, even more so due to the COVID-19 pandemic, by launching the Kairos Clubhouse—a live, interactive two-way show that connects individuals and groups through dance and creativity. It reaches a network of senior centers and organizations who serve people with disabilities across the state of Minnesota, and beyond. This innovative platform has allowed us to continue building our community and enabled people of all ages and abilities to experience the joy of movement, even remotely.

Intergenerational work and movement are deeply rooted in my lifelong passion for dance, coupled with my family background and experiences that emphasized the importance of intercultural and intergenerational connections. As such, Kairos Alive! has become a vessel for me to create transformative experiences where people from diverse backgrounds and ages can come together, move, and connect through the universal language of dance. Our work continues to evolve, reflecting our commitment to fostering inclusive and participatory art-making experiences that promote healing and well-being for all.

As we move forward, we acknowledge that there is still much to learn about the profound bond between artists, creativity, healing, and practice. Our mission is to continue translating the benefits of intergenerational and intercultural engagement into practical, everyday life, making it accessible to people of all ages and backgrounds. Through dance and music, we strive to bring people alive and encourage them to move, connect, and thrive.

DANA GRIFFIN

Co-founder and CEO, Eldera

eldera.ai

Unlocking the time and wisdom of older adults as a new natural resource for all generations to thrive.

"We can replace loneliness with a more joyful and healthy global village."

I was raised by my grandparents in Transylvania and Romania, and I've surrounded myself with older adults my entire life. A third of my friends are between their sixties and nineties. I rely on them to help me make decisions about my life, from career moves to investment matters, to health and relationships. That's how I navigate my life.

When one of my closest elder mentors passed away from brain cancer, I realized that the relationship we had was incredibly meaningful and symbiotic, and that I wanted to use technology to allow every child to have someone like my mentor in their lives. A career focused on aging led me to create Eldera, which stands for bringing forth the Era of the Elder.

Our vision is to radically, and globally, change the way we view aging, and improve the role of older adults in society. When we look at the world, we see generations separated in a way that hurts everyone. We see ageism, and eldercare is often viewed as a liability. Eldera's view of older adults is just the opposite. Our elders are assets. They teach us, nurture us, and help build intergenerational bonds that are joyful and engaging for every child and parent who is part of our program.

Using technology, Eldera connects vetted older adults (60-plus) with children (ages five to eighteen) via weekly virtual conversations and activities. Open to anyone who can benefit from this program, matches are made, regardless of geography, demographic factors, or mobility. There are a billion people over the age of sixty in the world today. In the years ahead, this number will double. Meanwhile, we have huge global challenges that need new resources, so we need to make better use of our incredible pool of older adults. The idea of bringing the old and young together is as long-standing as our species. Older adults have two of the most valuable resources on earth: time and wisdom.

The Centers for Disease Control and Prevention reported in 2022 that 71% of teenagers feel lonesome and isolated, which unleashed a global loneliness epidemic. Meanwhile, a third of our elders are lonely, with the World Health Organization reporting that this percentage increases to 50% for seniors over eighty. Loneliness is not just the domain of older adults. Nations are struggling to create solutions with both the United Kingdom and Japan founding governmental arms called 'loneliness ministries' to address this widespread problem.

Eldera believes that the solution lies in reuniting the generations. Older adults benefit from an increased sense of purpose and community, supporting healthy longevity, and productivity in society. Youths in intergenerational relationships gain resilience and social-emotional skills, while their parents gain partners in bringing their children's potential to life. Because evolutions in technology allow us to connect generations in a safe and nurturing environment that is beneficial to both, we can replace loneliness with a more joyful and healthy global village.

The Eldera program began just two weeks after New York schools closed due to the COVID-19 pandemic. We could not have imagined back then where we would be today. We have mentors in all fifty states and young participants from twenty-seven different countries. We've forged relationships with school boards and partnered with two of the top three school districts in the United States to offer Eldera as an after-school social and emotional program.

These collaborations are bolstered by the published study of Harvard University Center on the Developing Child. The study shows that building one-on-one relationships with non-parental adults fosters resilience in children and youth. In addition, research by the AARP Foundation Experience Corps, published in partnership with the National Institutes of Health and John Hopkins University, states that intergenerational relationships also improve academic outcomes.

Besides the scientific and emotional health advantages, participants have fun. Our members and mentors state unanimously that the number one benefit they get from joining Eldera is greater joy. Older adults look forward to their interactions with younger people and tell us that their young mentees never miss a session. Children say that they have each made a friend who is interested in their ideas, and shows up for them week after week. Meanwhile, parents notice improved confidence and scholastic achievements in their children. Additionally, teachers note an increase in the social-emotional skills of the young participants. This bonding shows us that we're making a difference. As we move forward, we plan to monitor these accomplishments, measure success, and watch for further growth in this interesting virtual environment.

MICHAEL HEBB

Founder, Generations Over Dinner

generationsoverdinner.com

A dinner party challenge to gather multiple generations at the table.

"We believe that the solutions to many of our problems may be discovered by the simple action of convening multiple generations around a table to have significant and vulnerable conversations."

I grew up in a unique setting in an intergenerational family. My father was born during the Gold Rush in 1904 in a miner's shed in Dawson City, Canada's Yukon Territory. By the time I joined this world, he was already 72 years old. My parents were twenty-nine years apart in age and I had four half-siblings that, if all of them were alive today, would be 90, 87, 84, and 78. I'm 47 now, and I also have a brother three years older than me.

Having lived a full life, my father shared his wisdom with us. I also experienced the middle-aged anxiety of my mother and the various personality types and contributions offered by my brothers and sisters. My family life helped me to embrace age differences. I felt comfortable with people significantly older than me and often sought their companionship.

When my father became ill and died because of Alzheimer's complications, I needed support and guidance. Fortunately, from age 15 on, I had a series of extraordinary mentors that transformed my life. However, if I wasn't so generationally diverse in my upbringing, I might have been timid about accepting their help. The confidence given to me by these mentors, the promise that people saw in me, and the time and energy that they gifted me, allowed me to believe that I could do important things.

These early experiences led me to mentor others early in life. In high school, for example, I received training in a program for those naturally inclined to help other students. Ever since then, people looking for mentorship have shown up in my life. And I continue to have my own mentors, too.

Person-to-person communication is irreplaceable. Being in direct contact with others has a greater impact on us than anything we see in the news, watch on social media, or read in books. On the flip side, there are stereotypes painted across every generation, but it's more passionately focused on the old and the young. I started Generations Over Dinner as a device to combat these labels, and as a tool to encourage older and younger people to have meaningful conversations that explore engaging topics.

Generations Over Dinner was inspired by Chip Conley's work with Modern Elder Academy (MEA) and my own life experience and values. I admired what was happening at MEA with its programs and workshops to promote a healthy and vital second half of life while incorporating community and intergenerational ties.

A team of social leaders and advisors joined me in a think tank environment to create a social ritual that would amplify the core values of MEA with a short time investment, flexible enough to work in many settings. During our brainstorming sessions, we selected the dinner format to meet our goal. Using the established social practice of friends, family, and co-workers eating together, we named our initiative Generations Over Dinner because it exemplifies the world we want to live in. The challenge was to see how many generations we could bring to the table.

Generations Over Dinner is a free initiative open to everyone, and can run without facilitators or significant funding. People host their own live events or digital gatherings using dinner scripts and guidelines found on our website. We constructed three different topic areas: Love and Relationships, Purpose, and The Future. Each engaging topic has three different scripts to focus on, with five questions per script.

Dinner conversations start by having everyone honor an ancestor, someone who had a powerful impact on them. Stories open the heart of participants, young and old. Then we move to questions. One standard query is, "What stereotypes do you think people associate with your generation? From your own experience, which ones do you think are right or wrong?" These questions go a long way to initiating meaningful interaction.

Other discussion items are:

"What were your most significant failures and what did you learn from them?"

"When was the last time you changed your mind about something? What was it and how did it affect your life?"

"What are three aspects of your parent's personality that you have or would like to have? What are three traits you dislike?"

These, are just a few examples.

Each dinner concludes with a gratitude exercise where participants tell the person next to them something they admire or appreciate about them. The feedback that we've received from these gatherings include descriptors ranging from 'transformative' to 'a really wonderful time' to 'would love to do it again.'

Modeled after the project Death Over Dinner, which motivated over a million conversations since its launch ten years ago, we believe that Generations Over Dinner will also reach a million people, and even ten million or more around the world.

There are many positive results we've seen through these efforts, especially in the connection to community. For older adults, the most important outcome is a tonic for curiosity, which is an essential part of longevity and health span. As we age, we can get stuck in our own heads, and it can be a lonely place. The sense of isolation reported by approximately 70% of folks aged 60-plus is further complicated by ill health, anxiety, and stress. The discourse that we have around the table can reinvigorate the imagination, reawaken an interest in others, and help combat this loneliness.

These dinners offer elders an opportunity to interact with younger people rather than believing stereotypes that cause a disconnect, such as…

"Kids are always on their phones."

"Young people are impolite and impulsive."

"They don't know how to have conversations about important issues."

Older adults recognize that these generalizations are incorrect. They see the youth as representatives of the future, and become willing to give of themselves and share the insights they've learned.

The younger generations find that they have more in common with the elders than originally assumed. They relate to the feelings of isolation and express the desire to form that kind of meaningful connections. They may acknowledge that, yes, they are on their cell phones a lot, but they are also passionately engaged in social movements, deeply concerned about climate change, and are active in steps to address these and other issues. When it comes to engaging with people from older generations, the youth receive the implicit and explicit message, “It gets better. There’s a reason to persevere.”

There’s a great magnetism between the younger and older generations. You can feel it at the table where you have participants from those two spectrums. Overall, it creates an opportunity for empathy and mutual understanding. We believe that the solutions to many of our problems may be discovered by the simple action of convening multiple generations around a table to have significant and vulnerable conversations. There’s something life affirming about preserving these connections, being around human beings that have lived well and become a full expression of themselves.

Generations Over Dinner fosters connections. Connections offer hope, and hope makes a statement about a belief in the future. And, after all, who doesn’t love a good dinner party?

CHARLOTTE JAPP

Founder, Cirkel

cirkel.co

Connecting professionals across ages and career stages for mutual growth and co-mentorship.

"As the traditional career paths are evolving, intergenerational connections help bridge the gap between generations, enabling the transfer of knowledge, skills, and experiences."

My interest in intergenerational work was sparked by my upbringing and the relationship I had with my parents. Growing up in a household that valued interactions across generations, I naturally gravitated towards connecting with people of different ages, appreciating their unique perspectives. Whether it was family activities or gatherings for my parents' friends, my early exposure to the richness of diverse perspectives became the foundation for my interest in fostering intergenerational relationships.

As an adult, I moved back home after college and spent four years living with my parents. During this time, I observed the challenges of their careers as they aged out of the corporate world at around fifty, while I was simultaneously navigating my own entry into the workforce. Witnessing their journey, I pitched in with tech advice and supported their transition. They had to adapt and learn new skills, yet they had years of experience and knowledge that they shared with me. These mutual exchanges formed the foundation of my approach to intergenerational relationships, one based on equality, generosity, and shared knowledge.

Cirkel's evolution began when I recognized that many of my peers were working in environments dominated by young professionals, often prompting concerns about career progression after a certain age. Considering my parents' experiences, I grew worried about my own prospects. This realization motivated me to explore ways to recreate the intergenerational connections I had cherished at home.

As a result, Cirkel was launched in 2018 as an intergenerational networking event series. The aim was to bring together individuals across industries and ages, fostering open conversations in a relaxed setting (such as over coffee or cocktails). These engaging conversations encouraged discussions about work, life, and personal growth. As Cirkel evolved, we transitioned to a membership community that promoted deeper understanding across age gaps.

Despite challenges posed by the pandemic, our virtual membership expanded internationally, reaching more than ten countries. Cirkel has been instrumental in fostering both personal and professional growth across generations. Our approach ensures that intergenerational relationships are not one-sided but a dynamic exchange of insights and experiences.

Members have forged meaningful bonds, sparking personal and professional growth. For instance, the story of Kate and Leslie exemplifies the transformative power of intergenerational connections.

Kate, in her late twenties found inspiration from Leslie, a seasoned therapist in her late sixties, leading Kate to pursue a career in psychology. In turn, Kate's expertise in brand strategy helped Leslie establish herself as a thought leader.

These outcomes highlight the potential of intergenerational connections to drive personal development, professional growth, and bridge the gap between generations. Through my experiences, I've seen that they offer opportunities for continuous learning and growth, particularly in today's dynamic work environment. As the traditional career paths are evolving, intergenerational connections unite generations, enabling the transfer of knowledge, skills, and experiences. This not only enriches individuals' personal lives but also enhances their professional trajectories. Moreover, these connections challenge age-related stereotypes and promote understanding, leading to a more inclusive society.

My vision for the future is for intergenerational relationships to be seamlessly integrated into our everyday lives. Just as diverse friendships enrich our personal experiences, intergenerational connections can contribute to a more empathetic and interconnected society.

OLE KASSOW

Founder, Cycling Without Age

cyclingwithoutage.org

Building better lives through generosity and kindness.

"It starts with the generous act of taking one or two older or less-abled people out on a bike ride. It's a simple act that everyone can do."

I never imagined that a bike ride would lead to a global movement. It all began on the streets of Copenhagen, a city renowned for its love of cycling. Every morning, I cycled to work because I love cycling. One morning, I noticed an older man sitting on a bench in a sunny spot with his walking frame next to him. He sat there the next morning, and for the following two weeks. I could tell that he liked to spend time outside because he sported a very nice tan. He was always smiling, sometimes reading the newspaper, and always impeccably dressed in a casual country style. Talking to this ninety-seven-year-old gentleman, a nursing home resident, changed my life.

I have heard countless stories of people who have reluctantly had to give up cycling because they became afraid of being hit by a car door or crashing, and how much they miss the personal mobility and the freedom and the joy of cycling. I also had firsthand experience growing up with a father who battled multiple sclerosis (MS), witnessing the challenges faced by people with disabilities and limited mobility in urban environments. That fueled my determination to make a difference. I couldn't stand the thought of so many older adults and people with mobility issues like my dad had, feeling left out, forgotten, and lonely.

With all this in mind, one day I ventured to the local nursing home with a rented rickshaw. I realized it was a crazy idea, and that they would most likely kick me out. As I entered the nursing home, I was approached by this friendly-looking staff member. I said to her, "I'm a neighbor. I'm here to offer a ride to the residents." Now that could have been the end of the story. But the woman said to me, "Oh, that sounds like a great idea. Let me just check." Moments later, she reemerged with an older woman named Gertrude and declared, "Gertrude would love a ride."

I left in a rare spirit. The next day, I got a phone call from the manager of the nursing home. She wanted to know what I had done to Gertrude; all the other residents want to ride too. So, I rented the rickshaw again and I started offering bike rides to the residents in my spare time. It gave them a whole new mobility, and it gave me an insight into my city that I had never experienced. It was quite amazing, and I made lots of very unlikely friends. I felt like an explorer in uncharted territory.

That's how Cycling Without Age was born in 2012. I used to call it just "my crazy little idea." Get a rickshaw (similar to a three-wheeled bicycle), or bicycle with a really comfortable double seat at the front where two older adults or people with limited mobility can be seated, and then a 'pilot' pedaling the bike. I didn't really see any sort of bigger development of it, other than I wanted to see if I could make that difference to someone else.

Pretty soon Cycling Without Age was spreading to other cities in Denmark and then throughout the world. The positive feedback that we heard about the program was amazing. People who hadn't been talking for years started talking again. People suffering from dementia would lose their aggressions, and their spirits were lifted at the nursing home upon returning from their bike ride. Blind residents explained to the volunteers that, to them, cycling was all about smelling the flowers, hearing the birds, and feeling the wind in your hair. We're here to fight for people's wind in their hair.

The magic of Cycling Without Age lies not only in the physical act of cycling but also in the emotional connections it fosters. For the passengers, it's an opportunity to break free from the confines of their homes, reconnect with their communities, and engage in meaningful conversations with fellow cyclists. I still remember the emotional story of an older woman moved to tears by the sheer magnificence of her surroundings during one of our rides.

What astounds me the most is how bike rides can have such a profound impact on quality of life, both for the older adults and for volunteers. The magic of intergenerational bonds blossom through our program. The program has attracted a diverse group of volunteers. Approximately 40% of volunteers are young students between eighteen and twenty-five, and nearly 50% are close to retirement or already retired; the rest are people in between. Young volunteers get the chance to chat with, and learn from, older adults during bike rides, which leads to valuable intergenerational connections. The shared experience of cycling and storytelling creates lasting friendships and relationships, bridging generational gaps and fostering empathy and understanding. It's a beautiful dance of generations, and it fulfills a social need that society often overlooks.

One of the most significant effects of Cycling Without Age is addressing the pervasive issue of loneliness and isolation, a daunting challenge in today's society. We've created societies that segregate people rather than connect people. Well over 40% of the population is isolated and lonely, and that number is larger among older adults. It's amazing that we have allowed that to happen. Loneliness is a silent epidemic, and our bike rides aim to alleviate this burden. It is a testament to the power of human connection, delivered through a leisurely bike ride.

Cycling Without Age's guiding principles are generosity, slowness, storytelling, relationship, and without age. These principles serve as our guiding stars, reminding us that even the simplest acts of kindness can bridge generations and bring joy beyond measure.

1. **Generosity:** It reflects the core of volunteerism and the desire to make a positive difference in someone else's life. Studies have shown that people who are witnesses to acts of kindness feel an emotional elevation.
2. **Slowness:** Emphasizes the importance of taking one's time and creating opportunities for meaningful interactions during bike rides.
3. **Storytelling:** Acknowledges the power of sharing stories, which helps in bonding, making friendships, and understanding one another.
4. **Relationship:** Highlights the significance of building strong connections between people of different ages.
5. **Without Age:** Embraces the idea that age should not be a barrier to forming connections, learning, and growing together.

Cycling Without Age has taught me that beauty and joy can be constants in life, even as we age. The simple act of inviting someone, whether a neighbor or a stranger, on a journey through our cities and landscapes can create a world of difference. It's all about fostering relationships and celebrating a world where age doesn't matter, something we cherish deeply. We break free from societal norms that segregate individuals based on age and emphasize that intergenerational interactions enrich lives and broaden perspectives.

Today, our initiative has spread to over 3,000 chapters worldwide, with approximately 20,000 active volunteers—a testament to the incredible impact of this movement. As we continue to grow, I am filled with hope that our wheels will pave the way for more age-diverse communities worldwide, one bike ride at a time.

ELLY KATZ

Executive Director and Founder, Sages & Seekers

sagesandseekers.org

Working to develop empathy while combating social isolation and ageism.

"When stereotypes are shattered, curiosity develops. A curiosity of what different people with different perspectives can bring to the table. This is when we can bridge our differences and create social change."

I was listening to a National Public Radio speaker discuss the state of the planet while driving my sixteen-year-old son to school. Before he exited the car, my son addressed the topic by calling it an 'apocalypse'. I thought, "Wow. This is not good."

I continued to listen to the broadcast. The speaker said that if everyone chose to address something that they were passionate about, we could turn the world around. I thought to myself, "Well, I hope someone's listening to this because I don't have time to do that." But the speaker's words lingered, and I asked myself, "What am I passionate about?"

I decided that if I was going to do something important, it would be around the issue of ageism and social isolation. It's no secret that ageism is rampant today, and that goes both ways with negative stereotypes about older adults as well as teens. I also recognized a growing epidemic in America, older adults and teens are the two most isolated groups in our society. According to a meta-analysis, a lack of social connection heightens health risks as much as smoking fifteen cigarettes a day or having an alcohol use disorder. Back at home, I pulled out my laptop and started writing down my ideas. I wondered, *how can I make a difference?* Those ideas were the genesis for Sages & Seekers, a nonprofit program with an overarching goal to develop empathy, diminish ageism, and reduce social isolation among elders and young adults, while fostering connections and meaningful relationships.

Our participants are comprised of Sages (older adults age 60-plus) and Seekers (teens and young adults ages 15-24). We begin that process by creating co-generational communities. We enroll teens and elders in our evidence-based, eight-week programs. It is a gathering of generations where old and young come together as equals to share their lives as a community, as well as one-on-one. During those eight weeks we look at the human experiences shared by all of us—our hopes, fears, successes, failures—all the experiences of being human. This deep dive into the human condition develops empathy, which in turn lays the groundwork for connection. That connection creates a sense of belonging. And when you belong, you care—you want to create a better life for yourself and your community.

Weekly meetings, either in-person or online, last for about an hour. The first week focuses on shattering stereotypes, allowing both the Sages and the Seekers to see beyond age-based assumptions. We sit in a big circle, or as a virtual group, allowing older adults (the Sages) to see that the students (the Seekers) are not these insensitive young people. And vice versa. We ask questions like, "Has anyone ever run a red light? Have you been skinny dipping? Have you participated in a public protest?" The participants, young and old begin to recognize that human connection transcends age.

During the second week, rotating group discussions introduce students and older adults to one other. Then the Seekers have 'speed dates' to select a Sage that they will work with in the coming weeks via one-on-one conversations. Team members choose the topics, and discuss anything as long as both are comfortable. It is also their choice to say, "I don't want to talk about that." Over the sessions, they explore a myriad of subjects ranging from sex to careers, to illness and dying, to failure and triumphs.

To conclude the program, the Seekers write tributes to their Sages. I tell them, "Do not write your Sages' histories because they already know their own stories. Write about how their sharing has impacted your life." The students read their tributes in front of everyone, creating a moving and meaningful experience. In the final week, a debriefing session provides an opportunity for reflection on what surprised the Sages and Seekers most about one another.

Our program is thriving across the United States in schools and universities (both public and private), senior community centers, Lifelong Learning institutes, and programs in low-income areas. We have served over 6,000 participants from a wide variety of genders, races, and socio-economic backgrounds. Leveraging technology, we transcend physical borders and create virtual connections, fostering relationships across global sites like Australia, Argentina, and Columbia. Through these multicultural and intergenerational connections, we aim to strengthen the bonds of humanity.

There are many benefits of this intergenerational program. A University of Southern California study funded by the National Endowment for the Arts, as well as a study funded by the Templeton Foundation, support our program model and positive outcomes regarding adolescent values, engagement, social-emotional skills, confidence, and well-being. But perhaps the best recommendation is by the participants themselves. Both generations are searching for meaning and relevance in their lives, grappling with a common struggle against feelings of loneliness, a sense of not fitting in, or being marginalized. They share concerns surrounding concepts such as independence, self-determination, and staying current in a rapidly changing world.

The elder Sages feel relevant as they learn to understand the inner workings of a teen. They also feel valued, and develop relationships, share life experiences, and provide guidance to the next generation. Interactions with their Seeker partners may cause them to review their lives from a different perspective, yet recognize common feelings and thoughts that occur irrespective of age.

For the Seekers, the number one positive outcome is a greater sense of purpose, a payoff during the current mental health crisis. Interacting with older adults helps them break free from societal labels and gain a broader perspective on life. They develop social-emotional skills, including empathy, through their bond with a Sage. In addition, changes in their perception reflect a higher well-being and an awareness that often creates a greater interest in civic engagement.

When stereotypes are shattered, curiosity develops. A curiosity of what different people with different perspectives can bring to the table. This is when we can bridge our differences and create social change so we can address the important issues facing humanity today.

NICOLE KENNEY, M.P.P.

Founder, Hey Auntie!™

heyauntie.io

Hey Auntie!™ is a cross-generational digital platform and community facilitating connections for Black women to learn the rules, gain the tools and build the networks to thrive at home, work, and everywhere in between.

"Everyone needs support and peace of mind, regardless of age."

I grew up in an intergenerational environment with many 'aunties': my mother's sister, friends, cousins, coworkers, and women from my church. Yet, despite being surrounded by such a loving community, when I became ill from stress in my early thirties, I believed that I needed to act strong, cope on my own, and hold my thoughts and feelings inside. The truth is, it's easy to lose sight of the importance of community. I embraced the popularized individualistic mindset of 'do it yourself' and believed community, while important, was a luxury and not a lifeline. And as a Black woman, I didn't know what research now shows, namely that we experience higher stress levels due to racial and gender discrimination, that we lack culturally competent care, and we are less likely to seek support. (Collier et al., 2019) Looking back, this was me. Hopeless, I disconnected. And I suffered in silence.

My family discerned I needed support and came to visit me. That's one of the many beautiful gifts of community. When you do not have the strength to seek help, help finds you. My auntie, Dr. Deborah Darlene Roebuck, a women's health and public health expert was also in tow. She created a compassionate atmosphere that allowed me to share what I was experiencing. Her stories validated my experiences and provided guidance, support, and tools to survive and thrive despite being doubted, dismissed, and misunderstood. Most important, she reminded me that I come from a rich legacy of people whose strength lies in knowing that our mindset is always our mind to set.

In our history, as Black folks, especially Black women, we come from a rich legacy of support systems. The term 'auntie' extends back hundreds of years ago in West Africa. An auntie is defined as a woman who sees every child, not just her biological ones, as her child. This cultural legacy would be an emotional and social support system to generations of enslaved people who endured the cruelty of slavery in America, as so many families were split apart. This social network continues to promote the health and well-being of Black communities to this day.

Over time, as I experienced life with more older women, my network continued to expand with aunties. Initially, I thought an auntie was a specific age and life stage. This mindset was turned entirely on its head when I started teaching wellness classes at my childhood YMCA and became a personal trainer. Surprisingly, most of my class attendees and clients were women over sixty. These women were excited to learn strength training and nutrition habits from me. I had the privilege to walk alongside them, challenging them and watching them grow. They trusted me for advice, encouragement, and support, often within the realm of fitness and many times outside of it.

This moment taught me an important lesson: in every age and life stage, there are opportunities when you will be '*auntieing*' and opportunities where you will need to be '*auntied.*'

Being in a community with aunties also taught me the wisdom of valuing my time and being a good steward of my gifts and talents. I began to ask myself, "How can I make decisions now that I'll be proud of when I'm 80?" I decided to pursue a career consisting of purpose-driven social impact work. I created a consultancy where we design and implement innovative strategies, communications, and programs to advance racial, gender, and economic equity in businesses, their products, and the communities they serve.

Hey Auntie!™ emerged from my work, and offered diverse opportunities to serve my community, and share my own lived experiences. We are a cross-generational digital platform and community, facilitating connections for Black women to learn the rules, gain the tools and build the networks to thrive at home, work, and everywhere in between. We use the cultural legacy of the auntie as a framework to create a digitized space to foster connectivity and deliver social and emotional support. By employing this familiar approach, we can help weaken barriers and strengthen protective factors to empower Black women to seek help and live whole, productive, and healthy lives today, and for future generations.

At Hey Auntie!™, we've learned we need diverse connection styles depending on our season in life. We currently connect women in four primary ways on our platform: 1. Lela's Corners, which are small gatherings for peer-to-peer support around a specific issue or topic; 2. The Porch, which are large gatherings with an issue expert; 3. Auntie x Auntee, which is our 1:1 Matching Service where we pair a more experienced woman (an auntie) with a less experienced woman navigating a similar season (auntee); and 4. Community Aunties!, where women volunteer their expertise to support a nonprofit or community-based initiative. Ultimately, I envision Hey Auntie!™ in workplaces, academia, and healthcare institutions, driving policies and systems change to improve the health and well-being of Black women.

I'm often asked, "What's the best advice I receive from aunties?" What I hear the most is, "Be kind." In our culture, especially today, it's easy to get offended, think the worst, and assume something's a personal attack. An auntie once told me, "Be slow to take offense." You don't know what someone's going through. Some folks will express it, and others will suppress it. If you can share a kind word, do so because it can make the most significant difference in someone's day. Learning to be slow to offense is not always the easiest advice to receive. But, it has been the most transformational when practiced. It has also taught me the importance of humility, healthy conflict resolution, feedback, and correction, especially if you desire deep and long-term meaningful connections.

Today, it may seem millennials and Gen Zers are the generation that need support and peace of mind. Yes, we talk about it more. But being in cross-generational communities has taught me these needs exist across all ages and life stages. So, whether you are 19 or 91, ask yourself, "How can I value someone today? How can I love someone today? How can I support someone today?" Aunties have taught me that love, value, and support are universal languages.

Source:

Collier, Andrea and Bigger, Alana. "How Stress Impacts Black Women and Tips to Take Control." Healthline.com. September 25, 2019. https://bit.ly/3Q4FMoJ

MARJ KLEINMAN

Founder, Stoop Stories

stoopstories.com

Stoop Stories™ is a documentary storytelling project designed to connect, support, and celebrate our NYC neighbors, especially those hardest hit by the pandemic and systemic inequities.

"We honor generations of New Yorkers, past and present, who rejoice and take refuge in stoop culture."

The iconic stoops of New York have always brought New Yorkers together. It's where families make memories, youth hang out, and elders keep watch. In recent years, stoop life has eroded, particularly in gentrified neighborhoods with newcomers who don't know what it's all about. Safe and thriving communities are ones in which neighbors know each other, and care about each other's well-being.

During the 2020 lockdown, our stoops became our sanity and our solidarity. Some days, our stoops were our only connection to the outside world and I, myself, felt very lonely. That inspired me to venture out for a solo photographic series, visiting neighbors' stoops from the safe sidewalk. I explored my immediate area to create their portraits and hear how they were coping with COVID-19. I was able to see and hear familiar neighbors on a deeper level and get to know many I had never met. By creating colorful, vibrant environmental portraiture, I told a story of how the subject is grounded in a space—their stoop, their block, and their neighborhood. These portraits balanced authenticity and struggle with joy and upliftment. During lockdown, it felt urgent to document these stories. At age 50, I had found my life's work and the legacy I want to leave behind.

As a lifelong Brooklynite still residing in my childhood brownstone, I've spent countless hours sitting on its stoop, watching the world go by. In addition to being a visual storyteller, I was a writer and content producer specializing in children's educational media for twenty-five years. My academic background includes a Master of Arts in Educational Psychology from New York University and a Bachelor of Science in Theater Management from Emerson College. I've had the pleasure of teaching theater to kids and photography to adults. At home, I'm a proud mom to a feisty black cat named Blackberry who keeps me on my toes.

The concept of 'Stoop Stories' first came to me in 2011. I embarked on a project to interview my father, our friends, and neighbors right on their neighborhood stoops, aiming to preserve our shared stories. However, like many creative endeavors, this project was initially set aside. Fast forward to the onset of the 2020 lockdown, when isolation became a universal experience. During this time, I was living alone and in quarantine. As a photographer, I felt compelled to connect with others in some way, so I decided to venture out and take family portraits. This initiative quickly evolved into a larger project of documenting families' experiences during the COVID-19 pandemic, starting solo in Brooklyn and gradually expanding across New York City with a diverse collective of storytellers.

Since April 2020, we have collected and shared hundreds of these poignant stories, from families, essential workers, small business owners, activists, and artists throughout the five boroughs of New York City. Since not everyone has a stoop, we like to say, "A stoop is a state of mind." With that in mind, we visited sidewalks, storefronts, fire escapes, New York City Housing Authority (NYCHA) houses, the red steps in Times Square and the grand stairway of Brooklyn Borough Hall. We also hosted exhibits, including a three-floor show at the Brooklyn Children's Museum that featured an eleven-year-old storyteller and a makeshift stoop where families could pose for 'stoopies' (stoop selfies).

I first got involved with intergenerational content through my work in children's digital media at Sesame Workshop and PBS Kids. We were looking for ways to connect young children with their parents, grandparents, or caregivers through 'co-viewing' and 'co-play,' particularly for grandparents who weren't in the immediate vicinity. This wasn't merely about entertainment; it was a shared learning experience, rich with dialogue and social interaction that transcended the simplicity of the games themselves.

Last year, Stoop Stories began exploring intergenerational work through a series of short films and workshops between youth and neighborhood elders. These cross-generational duos shared life experiences, connecting in times of isolation and revitalizing a tradition that seemed to be ebbing away. We fostered these connections through workshops that preceded the filming. These sessions were designed to organically source stories and identify participants for the films. We found that the workshops helped build genuine bonds and trust, the foundation for the authentic conversations that would later unfold on camera. They weren't just about preserving stories; they were creating new ones.

With an initial grant from the Brooklyn Arts Council, we developed a pilot 'stoop chat' film featuring 'Harmonica Jimmy' and his friend

Shanaya, who met at our intergenerational workshops with Heights & Hills this summer. As these two bonded, they discovered a shared love of poetry, music, and street games.

Upon reflecting on her experience being a part of the film, Shanaya says, "The film definitely gives me more appreciation for all the hard work it takes to create a project within your community, trying to uplift people, trying to bring light toward situations that may not be exposed in the media. I'm hoping that the film opens people up to being a bit more kind and less judgmental toward others because you never know what anyone has battled. There are people in this world that are good, and you can overcome challenges and not be brought down by the things that you've encountered that may not be so nice."

'Harmonica Jimmy' says, "Most of all, I enjoyed connecting deeper with Shanaya, getting to know her a little more, and I really want to stay in her life. I text her poems every day now. Everybody you meet is not just a person passing by, they're a doorway to an entire world. This is a story of what connects Shanaya with me: resilience, poetry, music—it's about sharing one's spirit."

The film premiered at the Heights & Hills Center for Successful Aging and was attended by more than sixty people ranging from age 4 to 84. After viewing our two short films, participants engaged in a lively discussion about creating community together.

From the workshops to the films, there was this unmistakable sense of mutual respect and affection. Older adults felt heard, their lives witnessed, while the youth discovered new perspectives on community and history. The workshops were particularly moving; watching the participants choose their partners, seeing friendships bloom, and witnessing their eagerness to maintain these bonds post-workshop was nothing short of inspirational. Our goal extended beyond merely documenting these interactions. We wanted to inspire action, to encourage others to stop and chat with their neighbors, to build those crucial connections that foster a caring community.

Through multigenerational storytelling, we are preserving cultural legacies and reducing isolation, connecting elders and youth at a time when both groups are in severe need of connection. We are deeply committed to documenting the stories of neighborhood elders who have witnessed the changing neighborhood from their stoops, and have much to share with younger generations.

The call to action is twofold: first, to motivate individuals to engage in their own 'Stoop Chats,' fostering neighborly bonds, and second, to encourage the sharing of these intimate moments with a wider audience through our platform.

In essence, Stoop Stories has become more than a project. It has transformed into a full organization whose mission is to reignite community spirit, foster a sense of belonging and compassion with those who are similar and different from us. Our key goals are to help increase feelings of belonging and joy, reduce loneliness, and bring multigenerational communities together to support and celebrate each other. By helping neighbors create and share their own authentic stories, we honor and celebrate their lives. In this time of uncertainty, the stoops of New York have reminded us that, amidst the ebb and flow of city life, human connection endures, thrives, and stands resilient.

MARLENE KRASTOVITSKY

Co-Chair and Campaign Director, EveryAGE Counts

everyagecounts.org.au

Creating a society where every person is valued, connected and respected, regardless of age and health.

"The EveryAGE Counts team invites you to address ageism within and through your organization as a member of the EveryAGE Counts coalition."

I was fortunate enough to be the Director of the *Willing to Work National Inquiry* with the Australian Human Rights Commission. I was working with the late Susan Ryan AO, Australia's first Age Discrimination Commissioner. The Australian Government asked Susan to do an Inquiry into employment discrimination against older people and people with disability and to make recommendations for reform. (AHRC, 2016)

We travelled around Australia hearing countless heartbreaking stories of discrimination, ageism and ableism. These attitudes and practices were effectively locking people out of work and having devastating impacts on their lives and the lives of their families and communities. The injustice of it. What a waste! I heard repeatedly how pervasive, unchallenged, and invisible stereotypes, assumptions, and prejudices were leading to discriminatory behaviors. Ageism and ableism also have profound intergenerational effects.

I am also a daughter, a mother, and now, a grandmother. I never had the opportunity to know my grandparents, and always felt that this was a hole in my life. Sadly, my sons had limited opportunity to know their grandparents, but what was available to them was highly valued. Now, I have the great gift of being a grandmother, and I can experience first-hand the beauty of these relationships. I feel very fortunate.

We need to build intergenerational solidarity. Stereotyping older and younger people is not new. It is a human characteristic to form groups that form opinions about other groups. But what is new today is the use of generational categories like 'baby boomer' and 'Generation X' or 'Y' or 'Z.' Created as a marketing tool, these labels stay with age cohorts throughout their lives, unlike traditional labels, such as 'older,' 'younger,' 'teen,' etc., that represent the life stages through which people progress. They convey the idea that a person will always remain a 'boomer' or 'millennial,' and that all members of that group are identical and share particular values, aspirations and attitudes.

These generational categories are used today by some politicians in media and in public discourse. They contribute to narratives of disdain, division, and devaluing. However, these generalized labels do not reflect the experience or views of most Australians who live in intergenerational communities, especially within the family. Indeed, intergenerational connection and solidarity have been an under-reported feature of Australia's collective response to COVID-19.

Labelling a whole age cohort as the same is unhelpful. Marginal differences in behaviors and preferences between different age groups have been exaggerated into defining characteristics. Furthermore, there are much larger differences and inequalities between members within any given age cohort according to their gender, income, wealth, ethnicity, health status, and many other characteristics than between people of similar social status and identifications of different ages.

An ageing society, framed only as a series of challenges and deficits, with no countervailing analysis of the opportunities provided by demographic change, has fueled divisive rhetoric about intergenerational warfare.

We need a new narrative—a positive narrative that articulates the common interest of older and younger people. We need to foster a whole life course well-being for current and future generations, and intergenerational well-being, solidarity, and equality, now and in the future.

This requires, as a first step, abandoning the divisive, dehumanizing language of 'boomers' and 'millennials.' The old descriptions still work—children, teenagers, young people, middle-aged, older people. Evoking life stages rather than assigning labels that follow you through life allows for building stronger connections.

Ageism is rife in Australia, and it has devastating impacts. Ageism is stereotyping, discrimination or mistreatment based on age. Ageism fuels division by framing people as 'other.' Ageism is not benign or harmless. It is highly tolerated and often hidden. Ageism can also deny society the enormous range of benefits that can flow, economically and socially, from the full participation of people of all ages.

EveryAGE Counts is changing all that. EveryAGE Counts is Australia's national coalition and grassroots movement to end ageism. Our vision is a society where every person is valued, connected and respected, regardless of age. Our growing and diverse supporter base and coalition of organizations is spearheading a social movement with an ambitious agenda: to dismantle ageism.

While ageism can affect anyone of any age, the EveryAGE Counts campaign addresses ageism relating to older people because of its deeply damaging impact on this group of people. Having said that, we know from research that intergenerational connection reduces the extent to which people hold ageist views, so strengthening intergenerational solidarity is important. EveryAGE Counts does not support divisive intergenerational conflict or rhetoric that pits generations against each other. We aim to find a positive narrative that articulates the common interests of older and younger people. Well-structured and evidence-based intergenerational programs which bring people together across different life stages in meaningful exchange is an important strategy, as research tells us that intergenerational contact reduces the likelihood of holding ageist views.

Source:

Australian Human Rights Commission. "Willing to Work: National Inquiry into Employment Discrimination." May 2, 2016. https://bit.ly/4d5rNZQ

DR. ROGER LANDRY, MD, MPH

Presenter & Author of Live Long, Die Short: A Guide to Authentic Health & Successful Aging Owner & Founder of Bright Side of Longevity & Masterpiece

livelongdieshort.com

Empowering individuals and communities to reach their full potential.

"We have embraced the mission to inspire and cultivate individual growth, resilience and purposeful longevity, with a vision of meeting individuals at every stage of life."

My journey in the field of preventive medicine and healthy aging began in the Air Force, where I was entrusted with the health of pilots operating in high-risk environments. This experience was not only about keeping them physically fit but also about understanding their unique challenges and lifestyles. I recall working with a range of pilots, including test pilots and astronauts, at Edwards Air Force Base. One of my most memorable experiences was meeting Chuck Yeager, the first person to break the sound barrier. These interactions with extraordinary individuals like Yeager shaped my understanding of health and resilience.

After my twenty-three years of military service, I transitioned to a healthcare system in Pennsylvania. My role was to enhance preventive capabilities across the system. I remember saying, "I worked with people who were very healthy pilots and tried to keep them that way." This phase of my career underscored the importance of preventive measures in healthcare. However, I soon realized the systemic focus on revenue conflicted with my preventive approach. This led me to explore other avenues where I could apply my preventive medicine philosophy more effectively.

Around this time, my brother, who was involved with the MacArthur Foundation's ten-year study on successful aging, reached out to me. He proposed applying the study's findings, particularly the idea that lifestyle is a key determinant of how we age. This led to a collaboration with Dr. Robert L. Kahn, Ph.D., another lead investigator from the MacArthur Study and author of the book *Successful Aging*. Together, we discussed, and eventually started, Masterpiece Living, an organization that partnered with over 150 retirement communities, aiming to change the culture of aging. We wanted communities to realize that so much more is possible as we age. We emphasized empowering individuals and communities to adopt healthier lifestyles for better longevity.

As we worked through these partnerships, we emphasized training and resource provision, tailoring our approach to enhance the cultural and possibility aspects of senior living communities. Over two decades, we witnessed significant growth and increased investment in these ideals. When the COVID-19 pandemic hit, it brought new challenges and a shift in approach. During this period, Masterpiece Living underwent a change in leadership, and we began to pivot toward a content-based strategy. We developed a holistic content approach centered around a lifestyle profile. This profile provided individuals with a personalized dashboard reflecting their physical, intellectual, social, and spiritual well-being. The content we offered was tiered at different levels, from beginner to master, and predominantly online.

With a new direction, Masterpiece Living became simply, *Masterpiece*.

At this time, I acquired this content platform and transformed *Masterpiece* into a comprehensive program under my new company, Bright Side of Longevity. Brightside of Longevity (both my business and *The Bright Side of Longevity* podcast) was a natural progression for me, driven by my passion for preventive medicine. I realized the untapped potential in focusing on older adults, a demographic often overlooked in preventive health. Inspired by my brother and our collaborative insights, I dedicated myself to advancing preventive care in the context of aging, showing that a healthier, fuller life is achievable at any age.

Bright Side of Longevity, with *Masterpiece* content as a driving force, has embraced a mission to inspire and cultivate individual growth, resilience and purposeful longevity, with a vision of meeting individuals at every stage of life. We focus on holistic lifestyle as the major determinant in experiencing a healthy longevity, and we place high value on intergenerational engagement.

My commitment to this cause was further solidified when I authored *Live Long, Die Short: A Guide to Authentic Health and Successful Aging*. In writing this book, my goal was to reach a wider audience, especially those who might not be actively engaged in pursuing a healthier lifestyle. The book underscores my belief in the power of preventive medicine and the impact of lifestyle choices on aging.

One of the most impactful aspects of my work has been fostering intergenerational connections. I believe these connections are not just beneficial for older adults, but are essential for the health of our society. I often quote Dostoevsky: "The soul is healed by being with children." This quote resonates deeply with me, highlighting the mutual benefits of intergenerational interactions. These interactions bridge gaps between generations, fostering understanding and empathy.

Our perspective on life can be likened to two contrasting models. The first is the linear model, characterized by traditional aging and a steady decline, as if we are journeying alone with a finite time in each phase, constantly moving toward an inevitable end. By contrast, the second is the circular model, and it signifies a life that sustains engagement at every stage, akin to a shared journey with all living beings, with the potential for purposeful living and pursuits at every turn, fostering a connection with something greater than ourselves. *Masterpiece* wholeheartedly embraces the circular life concept, emphasizing intergenerational engagement and the renewal of purposeful living throughout the journey.

Intergenerational connection positively impacts health and well-being, while decreasing loneliness and depression in older adults, and builds empathy, character, and social skills in younger individuals. Research suggests that children require four to six supportive and attentive adults in their lives to thrive emotionally and socially. The research is still unclear on how many younger people older adults require, but it is clear there is a need.

In response to this need, *Masterpiece* created a ready-to-use campaign, 'Navigating Together,' which encourages meaningful intergenerational conversations. Designed for easy use within senior living communities, 'Navigating Together' bridges age gaps by sharing stories and gained wisdom that builds connection. This campaign provides a way for younger generations to share important events in their lives while encouraging the older generation to share their experiences in similar situations.

Different generational groups come together and field questions designed to engage both and stimulate conversation. For example, questions might include, "What world events do you worry most about?" "What is (was) dating like for you?" And, "What do (did) you worry most about at this age?" Questions vary depending on the demographics of the participants, but are carefully selected to matter, especially for the younger person.

'Navigating Together' grew out of four previous initiatives with *Masterpiece* senior living communities in which we were partnered. The first paired a community resident with a fifth-grade student from a nearby school. The goal was to have the older adult help the student with a learning challenge they were experiencing, such as reading, math, or writing. Once a week, for one hour, the common area in the community was populated with nearly thirty small card tables where pairs of people, with as much as a 70-year difference in age, sat and engaged.

What happened went way beyond the learning: friendships blossomed. Conversation evolved into discussions about life challenges. Residents were then invited to school and family events, and the fifth-grade class performed musical events at the community. Town newspapers made celebrities of the residents, and there was soon a waitlist of community members who wanted to participate. The initiative continued until these young students entered high school, but friendships persisted. This sparked more creative opportunities for both the community and the school to collaborate…all from this simple idea.

The second creative intergenerational approach involved a partner senior living community which offered free room and board to a Master's degree student at a local university. The student was studying music and agreed to play the violin regularly for the entire community. Once again, this arrangement went way beyond the added music. The young woman became an adopted celebrity and enjoyed deeper relationships with numerous residents and staff. Community leadership, residents and staff, and the student were unanimous in their satisfaction and praise for this unusual but highly successful initiative.

The third initiative was a pen pal program between residents of a *Masterpiece* community and a local elementary school. Fifth graders were connected with a volunteer senior living resident and exchanged letters…yes…pen and paper letters that were mailed. Teachers praised the program for its connection, literary value, and its historical aspects. Older adults hailed the opportunity for purpose, fun, and engagement.

Last, one other *Masterpiece* partner community joined forces with a local boy scout troop to regularly bake dog biscuits in the community's kitchen. The biscuits were brought to area animal shelters. Outcomes were readily identifiable within the boy scout troop, many of whom earned merit badges for civic engagement. Older adults praised the program as a much looked-forward to opportunity to connect with the young scouts…and dogs.

The 'Navigating Together' campaign was not just an exercise in conversation; it was a profound exploration of shared human experiences across generations. We field-tested this initiative and found that the conversations often continued long past the allocated time. Participants, both young and old, were eager to share their stories and listen to others. This campaign exemplified the power of communication in breaking down barriers and misconceptions between different age groups. The outcomes of these creative efforts were the positive effects on the participating older adults: engagement, purpose, friendships, and understanding.

My journey through the realms of preventive medicine, military healthcare, and healthy aging has been a testament to the belief that lifestyle choices play a crucial role in determining the quality of our later years. From working with esteemed pilots to pioneering programs like *Masterpiece*'s 'Navigating Together,' my focus has always been on enhancing life quality and fostering meaningful connections across generations.

MEG LAPORTE AND JORDAN EVANS

Co-Founders, Art Against Ageism

artagainstageism.org

Identifying, amplifying, and creating artistic endeavors that confront and address damaging stereotypes about age and aging.

"Through art and engagement, we aim to make ageism visible and foster understanding across generations."

Throughout modern history, art, in its many forms, has sought to address social issues, counter the harmful impact of mass media, and change our perspectives of the world. Artists have utilized visual, literary, musical, and performing arts to comment on, respond to, or advocate for change, and engage communities in dialogue and consciousness raising. We created Art Against Ageism as an alliance and media platform for the purpose of identifying, amplifying, and creating artistic endeavors that confront and tackle damaging stereotypes and misperceptions about age, older adults, and being older. We partner with organizations and other entities to create and implement strategic communication plans that use traditional, non-traditional, and other tactics to ensure the initiative's effectiveness and impact.

Meg LaPorte:

I've been involved in intergenerational work, primarily because of my background in the senior living and aging services field. I founded the *Age in America* blog (LaPorte, 2016) to help reframe perceptions of aging and older adults. This soon became my passion project as well as the foundation for my work in advocating for older adults and tackling ageism. Over the years, my work in this industry led me to an interest in fostering intergenerational connections.

It all began after I taught a course at the University of Maryland, Baltimore County in 2018, where Jordan was one of my students. The course focused on using art as a tool to combat ageism, and the subject matter resonated deeply with Jordan. Our collaboration started from there.

During the pandemic, we decided to activate our shared vision. Although our work predominantly revolves around senior living, we understand that these communities inherently involve multiple generations, sometimes up to five, working, living, and volunteering together. Therefore, our work has a natural intergenerational component because of the diverse demographics within senior living.

The positive outcomes we've observed from our intergenerational connections are significant. For example, we recently attended the American Society on Aging conference, where we set up 'Own Your Age' photo booths. People from various generations within the aging services field took part, holding up their ages via decorated signs and sharing their experiences on social media. This activity exemplified the power of intergenerational connections, as it allowed people of all ages to celebrate their own ages, learn from each other, challenge stereotypes, and foster a sense of belonging across generations.

Jordan Evans:

My journey into intergenerational work is deeply personal. I've always lived an intergenerational life, growing up with grandparents who were very close to me. My family had strong intergenerational relationships, which significantly shaped my perspective. I had older cousins, and my grandmother was the youngest of thirteen, so I was often surrounded by older family members. Life naturally presents us with intergenerational relationships if we pay attention. It's like the saying, "You don't see something until you're looking for it." Nursing homes, for instance, are often overlooked until you work in the industry, but once you do, you notice them everywhere.

One of the most significant positive outcomes of intergenerational relationships is the exchange of knowledge. Interacting with older generations allows you to be ignorant without embarrassment, which is often not the case when dealing with peers of the same age. Older individuals don't expect you to know everything, and are pleasantly surprised when you share your insights. It's a humbling experience for both parties involved.

Meg and I met during my college years when she was my professor. Our connection grew from there, and during the pandemic we both felt compelled to address how society was responding to COVID-19, particularly the way certain age groups were prioritized over others. Meg's passion, and her course on combating ageism using art, activated me, giving me the tools to pursue my passion for intergenerational relationships. We've been on this exciting journey together, continually learning and growing.

Our goal with Art Against Ageism is to promote age positivity and combat ageism through artistic activism. We use various mediums, such as murals and community art projects, to bring generations together and challenge societal perceptions of aging. Our vision extends to creating intergenerational communities within senior living and connecting different institutions, such as schools and aging services, to bridge generational gaps. Art Against Ageism exists not only to create and promote actions that tackle damaging stereotypes about age and aging in creative ways, but also to help others create their own campaigns that seek to raise awareness of, and dismantle, ageism. Through art and engagement, we aim to make ageism visible and foster understanding across generations.

Source:

LaPorte, Meg. Age in America. 2016. ageinamerica.blog

MARK L. MERIDY

Executive Director, DOROT, Inc.

dorotusa.org

Bringing the generations together for over 45 years.

"The word 'DOROT' is a Hebrew word that means 'generations,' and this concept has been at the heart of our organization since its establishment in 1976. DOROT was founded by recent graduates of Columbia University with a clear mission: to bridge generational gaps and serve not only the Jewish community, but the broader community as well."

I grew up in a family where community service held great importance. Our focus was always on helping those in need and making the world a better place in any way we could. I had a special connection with both my maternal grandmother and paternal grandfather, both of whom I found to be truly inspirational, albeit in very distinct ways. They were both lovely individuals.

During my high school years, our youth group initiated a community service project where we visited residents at a nursing home. We were simply dropped off at the nursing home with no preparation or guidance, and while many of my friends found the experience extremely uncomfortable, I cherished it. I had no trouble walking into those rooms and striking up conversations with the residents. This, along with the strong connection to my grandparents, marked the beginning of my lifelong affinity for older adults.

When I went off to college and moved into an apartment in downtown DC, I had the pleasure of living on the same floor as several older individuals. I would regularly check in on them, offer to accompany them to the store, and even run errands for them when the weather was bad. So, when I was thinking about what I wanted to do professionally, I decided that I would go into the nonprofit space, specifically the field of aging. It was just very natural for me.

Over the course of my career, I have worked at an Area Agency on Aging in Massachusetts where I served as the director of the home-care department and worked on a grant from the Administration on Aging to address transportation and mobility issues for older adults. I also played a role in constructing Section 202 housing for older adults. However, I noticed that these roles primarily focused on helping older adults live independently in the community, as per the focus of the Older Americans Act. What seemed to be missing was attention to helping them thrive in a society that heavily emphasizes youth. Many older adults, especially those who had retired, were left feeling lost and forgotten. Their social circles had dwindled as they aged, leaving them with fewer people to connect with.

It was during this time that a search firm approached me about heading an organization on the Upper West Side of Manhattan, even though my family and I were residing in Washington, DC, at the time. Although I hadn't previously heard of the organization, I was instantly drawn to its mission of bridging the generations and tackling the issues of social isolation and loneliness among older adults.

I've now been with DOROT since 2009, and I can confidently say it's the most rewarding job I've ever had. The impact our programs have on our participants is truly profound and incredibly gratifying. The word 'DOROT' is a Hebrew word that means 'generations,' and this concept has been at the heart of our organization since its establishment in 1976. DOROT was founded by recent graduates of Columbia University with a clear mission: to bridge generational gaps and serve not only the Jewish community, but the broader community as well. I take great pride in the fact that, while our organization is rooted in Jewish values that honor our elders, we extend our services to everyone in the community.

One of the unique characteristics of DOROT is our expansive definition of intergenerational programming. When most people think of intergenerational, they think of young people with older adults. And that certainly falls within DOROT's definition as well. However, we also consider a 45-year-old meeting with a 92-year-old as intergenerational.

At DOROT, we provide an opportunity for everyone to feel valued. Many of our older adults are isolated and alone and often feel invisible and forgotten. In some cases, they are simply unable to leave their home on a regular basis to engage in life-enhancing community activities. What we do is offer a chance for all participants to engage and interact with one another in a meaningful way. For some, this means coming to DOROT's main office to enjoy peer-to-peer and intergenerational activities. For others, this means welcoming volunteers of all ages into their home for social visits, technology coaching, errand support, birthday celebrations, and more. Additionally, our work at DOROT goes beyond simply bringing generations together; we also enable people to meet and learn from individuals they might never have had the opportunity to encounter otherwise. This is one of the truly beautiful aspects of the work we do at DOROT.

Allow me to share a touching story that reflects the essence of DOROT's work. This story takes us back in time, but it recently resurfaced when someone inquired about a photograph hanging in our DOROT office. The photograph captures a moment between a young man and an older adult. The young man is playing the cello, and they are both engrossed in sheet music. The older adult in this image was a Holocaust survivor, a man who had experienced immense hardship and loss. He had no family left, as they had all perished during the Holocaust, and he was battling profound depression and anxiety.

At that time, we had a program that partnered with Action Reconciliation Service for Peace (ARSP). This program provided young German volunteers with the opportunity to come to the United States and work with Jewish organizations as an alternative to military service. One of these volunteers, a young German named Christoph, was the cello player in the photograph.

Initially, the older gentleman, Arthur, had no interest in meeting Christoph. He was hesitant to connect with a young German whose grandfather had been in the Third Reich's army. However, a persistent social worker suggested they meet, highlighting Christoph's aspiration to become a cellist and Arthur's accomplished background in playing the cello.

Their first meeting was far from smooth with Arthur expressing his reservations. He even remarked, "If we were living fifty years ago, you would have killed me." Despite this rocky start, their relationship gradually transformed into a profound connection. Even after Christoph returned to Germany, he continued to stay in touch with Arthur until Arthur's death.

As time passed, Christoph got married and had a son. To honor the meaningful bond he shared with Arthur, Christoph named his son Arthur. This story is a testament to the extraordinary impact of genuine human connections. Such magical moments may not occur every day, but the approach DOROT takes in its weekly and monthly Friendly

Visiting programs can genuinely improve the quality of life for both the volunteers and the older adults we serve.

For many years, we've understood that the absence of social engagement and connections can lead to severe healthcare consequences. Over the past decade, research has further highlighted the devastating health impacts of social isolation and loneliness. Just last year, the US Surgeon General, Vivek Murthy, issued an unprecedented report, indicating that we are facing an epidemic of loneliness and social isolation not only in the United States but also globally. Our mission at DOROT is to provide older adults with a sense of purpose and the opportunity to remain socially engaged and connected within our community.

Our approach involves both peer-to-peer programming and a strong intergenerational focus. It's through this intergenerational lens that we accomplish our work. What sets DOROT apart is our deliberate and comprehensive approach. Unlike my junior high school experience, where we were simply dropped off at a nursing home and told to visit with the elderly residents, DOROT will never send volunteers into the homes of older adults without proper training and orientation. Also, we won't send volunteers of any age to make a home visit unless the older adult has been home assessed by a DOROT social worker. All our intergenerational programming is carefully planned, and we have a pedagogical approach that emphasizes mutual benefits for both older adults and young individuals.

Especially after the pandemic, people now have a much greater understanding and appreciation of the impact of isolation and loneliness. We are meticulous in creating an environment conducive to positive interactions. We place a strong emphasis on creating an equitable and respectful space for everyone involved. Both older and younger participants are given opportunities to establish mutual agreements, outlining how the program will be developed and implemented. For our teen and college internship programs, we empower young participants to take a leadership role in shaping the programs they will be involved in. They aren't just following a set path; they take ownership of their interactions with older adults.

We also work with older adults to set expectations: fostering active listening, empathy, patience, and the ability to collaborate within a supportive community marked by mutual respect. Simply bringing together older and younger people without this deliberate approach can often lead to negative outcomes.

One of our most successful and popular initiatives involves legacy projects, where older adults have the opportunity to share their life stories. These projects take various forms, including young people writing short stories about their older friends' life experiences, collaborating on art projects, or partnering with a film company to create legacy film projects. In the film projects, young participants learn to interview older adults, use cameras, film the interviews, and even edit them. We also conduct storytelling sessions where both younger and older individuals learn how to craft compelling stories with a beginning, middle, and end, developing a captivating narrative arc. Additionally, we engage in intergenerational art projects, and we offer a very successful and innovative intergenerational chess program. During the pandemic, our programs needed to shift from being in-person to all being online. Thankfully, we are now able to do both. One very successful program that we started as a result of the pandemic was GENuine Connections™, our exclusively online intergenerational community where teens and older adults enjoy cohort-based activities together; we offer three to four semesters each year.

Our intergenerational programs run year round, including internships, with extensive and intensive summer programs catering to high school and college students. These initiatives are all about fostering meaningful connections between generations. An impact report highlights the positive outcomes of our intergenerational programming. Young participants gain a deeper understanding of the challenges faced by older adults and learn the value of lived experiences, leading to a reduction in ageism. Many have been inspired to pursue careers in the field of aging or explore social work because of their experiences. For older adults, it provides a sense of purpose and renewed meaning in their lives, particularly if they have limited social connections. Moreover, our programs create a safe, judgment-free space where young individuals can be themselves, free from the pressures and expectations they may face in their peer groups and schools. This authenticity is a powerful and transformative outcome of our intergenerational work.

KEERTHANA PARAMASIVAM

Founder, GenLab Collective

genlabcosg.org

Bridging generations, empowering older adults.

"We provide a platform for people from different generations to share, learn and collaborate with the aim of bridging generation gaps in the longer term."

Growing up in Singapore, my personal experiences have shaped my interest for intergenerational work. I witnessed the struggles my grandmother endured with Alzheimer's and the resulting impact on my family, particularly on my mother and her sisters who took on caregiver roles. This made me deeply cognizant of the significance of health and well-being as we navigate the path of aging. It also struck me that while there was a lot of emphasis on youth mental health, the older generation seemed overlooked, at least from my perspective. My personal experiences, along with observing the mental health concerns of the older population during the COVID-19 period, notably increased suicide rates, drove me to champion their cause.

My initial involvement in intergenerational work was sparked by my participation in the "Youth Action Challenge" an initiative organized by the National Youth Council in Singapore during the COVID-19 pandemic. It commenced with facilitating Zoom sessions where older adults could display and share their wealth of skills and knowledge. This was a reflective response to the increasing mental health struggles witnessed among the older adults during these trying times.

In 2021, I founded GenLab Collective as a nonprofit ground-up initiative run by a team of youths where we aim to bridge the generation gap within our community. Through this, we also hope to offer a space for older adults to share their unique experiences, knowledge, and skills with the younger generations. The framework of GenLab Collective is innovatively designed to leverage the design thinking method, emphasizing co-creation in our programs and activities by offering a platform for diverse age groups to collaborate, connect, and co-create.

Traditionally, there's been a push for lifelong learning among older adults, but less thought has been given to how we might empower them. How do we offer platforms, opportunities, and tools that not only recognize but also celebrate their unique strengths and skillsets? During our initial discussions, it was clear that many older adults were eager to contribute to society—they wanted to share their skills and knowledge, but some lacked the right avenues to do so.

This is where GenLab Collective steps in. We're dedicated to providing older adults with enjoyable, innovative opportunities to present themselves and their capabilities. Through skill-sharing initiatives and broader community engagement, we aim to highlight our senior community's unique strengths. Moreover, we strive to foster intergenerational bonding, creating spaces where older and younger individuals can interact, leading to enriching exchanges of skills, knowledge, and life experiences.

One of our key flagship initiatives is GenNarrates, a storytelling program where youths partner with older adults to translate their stories and experiences into digital and interactive formats. By the end of the program, youths and older adults co-create the format and narrative in which they would like their stories and experiences to be presented.

The value of our intergenerational program is multifold. These initiatives don't just provide activities; they rebuild a sense of purpose, belonging, and community. Young people learn the art of empathy and communication, growing more comfortable and confident in engaging with older generations. Older adults often express a newfound joy in connecting with the youth, debunking their assumption that the younger generation is too preoccupied for such interactions. They find themselves learning and sharing, particularly absorbing digital and creative skills from the younger participants. It's a mutual discovery of value, breaking down preconceived barriers and enriching lives on both ends of the age spectrum.

Our core mission is to bridge the generational divide within Singapore, cultivating an inclusive community that honors every age. We harness the power of storytelling and active listening to unite people for collaborative creation, partnering with educational, corporate, and community groups to reinforce this vision. Our objectives are clear: facilitate deep intergenerational dialogue, provide platforms for mutual learning, preserve the stories of older adults, stimulate people's minds, and empower older adults to share their insights.

The work we do is not just about bridging the generation gap—it's about creating shared narratives, where every individual, young or old, is equally vital. Our efforts have rippled through the community. We're seeing a cultural shift, one that embraces all ages, fosters respect for each other's stories, and ultimately, knits a more inclusive society. In doing so, we're celebrating the unique contributions of all generations, weaving a social fabric where everyone, young and old, can thrive together. This is the heart of GenLab Collective—connecting generations, one story at a time.

FERNANDE RAINE

Founder, History Co:Lab

thehistorycolab.org

Innovating how students experience learning history so that they grow up empowered to take on the challenges of today and realize the opportunities of tomorrow.

"Young people as co-designers and co-creators bring a fresh perspective and ignite curiosity and inspiration, breaking stereotypes about their engagement and commitment to meaningful change."

My journey into intergenerational work was fueled by a blend of personal experiences and a strong desire for positive societal change. Growing up with a dual heritage—German and American—instilled in me a profound awareness of the consequences when democracy falters, as seen in Germany during the 1930s. This understanding ignited a lifelong commitment to ensuring such events never recurred, and that humanity progressed towards a brighter future.

My passion for history played a pivotal role in this journey. I viewed history not merely as a record of the past, but as a tool to shape the future. This perspective led me to extensively study history and recognize its significance in understanding one's role in crafting a better tomorrow.

During my student years, I was deeply engaged in democracy-related activities, and I vividly recall the sense of empowerment that defined that phase of my life. We, as students, ran organizations, campaigned for change, organized student governments, and participated in protests. These experiences reinforced my belief that individuals, regardless of age, possess the capacity to make a difference and usher in positive transformations.

Later, I transitioned into the realm of social entrepreneurship, working with organizations like Ashoka (ashoka.org), which aimed to empower every person to become a changemaker. This phase, focused on systemic change and creating fellowships, further solidified my commitment to driving societal progress.

I founded History Co:Lab intending to reshape history education to inspire young individuals to become critical, caring, and curious changemakers. The core challenge was to make history, often viewed as dull, relevant and engaging for young learners.

However, my perspective underwent a significant shift when I involved young people directly in the creative process. While attending a conference in India, I met a seventeen-year-old who passionately advocated for youth involvement in history education. His frustration with a tokenistic representation of youth voices in such events resonated with me. We decided to collaborate and created a youth-driven podcast as an experiment. The results were remarkable. The youth's unique perspective and enthusiasm breathed life into the project, making it engaging and authentic.

This experience convinced me that co-designing with young people yields exceptional results. They don't just need to be included at the end of the process; they should be co-creators from the beginning. The energy and innovation they bring to the table are unmatched.

Our organization, History Co:Lab, operates on multiple fronts to transform history education. We work with prominent foundations and institutions aiming to reshape the future of learning, ensuring that history and the humanities are considered as important as STEM subjects. During our design workshops, young people play a pivotal role in shaping the learning experiences of the future.

Additionally, we collaborate with community organizations and institutions, such as museums and libraries, to design learning experiences that ignite the curiosity and inspiration of young learners. Game-based experiences and interactive projects are some of the ways we engage with these institutions, always involving young people in the design process.

Our flagship project, the "UnTextbooked" (untextbooked.com) podcast, connects young people with renowned historians, changemakers, and journalists. Young podcasters select topics they are passionate about and interview experts, adding their unique perspective and asking probing questions. The podcast not only provides a platform for young voices but also demonstrates their ability to facilitate meaningful conversations.

The impact of our work is multi-faceted. First, it equips young people with the skills to become effective changemakers. They gain confidence in moderating high-profile conversations, interviewing experts, and asking insightful questions. Organizations now seek their participation, recognizing their potential to bridge generational gaps in discourse.

Second, the authenticity of young voices in our podcast has a profound effect on adult listeners. It challenges stereotypes about teenagers, highlighting their intelligence, curiosity, and passion for making a difference. Many adults find renewed hope and excitement in witnessing the commitment of young people to understanding complex issues, while also shaping their future.

Our work is not limited to young podcasters and listeners. We are actively working toward integrating our podcast into educational institutions, making it a part of the learning process. By doing so, we aim to redefine education as a series of transformative experiences that empower young individuals to thrive in a rapidly changing world.

My inspiration for intergenerational work emerged from a combination of personal experiences and a profound belief in the power of young people to shape the future. Through History Co:Lab, we strive to revolutionize history education, engage young learners, and bridge generational divides. Our journey is marked by a commitment to 'go big or go home' and to continue challenging the status quo to empower the changemakers of tomorrow.

SEAN-PIERRE REGIS

Duty Free Film, Director

dutyfreefilm.com

Duty Free is a film that follows the journey of a 75-year-old immigrant mother who gets fired without cause from her lifelong job as a hotel housekeeper. Her son takes her on a bucket-list adventure to reclaim her life. As she struggles to find work, he documents a story that uncovers the economic insecurity shaping not only her future, but that of an entire generation.

"Intergenerational connection isn't just about casual conversations or sharing past stories; it's about exploring who we are at our core, learning about ourselves through someone else's experiences."

My mother was always my best friend despite our 43-year age difference. However, it wasn't until she lost her job at age 75 that I truly understood that our bond was intergenerational. Filming her struggles to find work and accompanying her on a bucket-list adventure, I realized the immense value of our exchange of insights, support, and life experiences. This revelation inspired my film, *Duty Free*.

Duty Free tells the story of my mother, a single mom and hotel housekeeper in Boston who worked tirelessly until she was dismissed for her age. The film follows our adventure as she enjoys life adventures that she missed out on while working, such as skydiving and reuniting with her sister. But it also highlights a broader issue: the challenges faced by an aging population living longer with fewer resources.

Ageism and financial insecurity in America are pervasive. Older adults are often invisible in their communities, workplaces, and sometimes, within their own families. An estimated 25 million won't have enough money to get through retirement age. *Duty Free* examines ageism, the care crisis, and economic insecurity in America. Important questions we should all be asking are, "Who will care for and support our moms and dads? Our grandmothers and our grandfathers? Who will support us as we age?"

From my experience, intergenerational connections reveal the universality of our life paths. They break down age-related stereotypes and open doors to learning from the life stories of older generations, preparing us for similar issues. The beauty of these connections lies not just in shared joy, but also in navigating and overcoming misunderstandings and difficulties together, fostering a deep understanding of the human condition across age divides.

When I began this exploration, I grappled with the very real notion that we're all going to age. This is a universal truth we all share—the inevitability of growing older. Recognizing this, especially as a young person, opens up a profound understanding of our shared humanity. It makes you realize that the stereotypes and misconceptions we've learned about older people are often far from the truth. Embracing this understanding uncovers beauty in the most unexpected places.

This journey of discovery involves delving deep into the human condition through the experiences of someone older. It's about understanding heartbreak from someone who's lived through it, maybe once, or even several times. It's about recognizing that, like them, we will all need care at some point. We are all on this same path as human beings, encountering problems and facing life's obstacles.

Sharing these conversations has been invaluable. Discussions about love, about the challenging decisions my mom had to make, which we explored in the film, have been enlightening. Learning from her, from her 'heart stuff,' has been like receiving a manual on how to navigate similar life situations. Opening myself up to this intergenerational connection has given me a preview of the paths life might take. Now, I feel more secure. The unknown doesn't seem as daunting, frightening, or insurmountable. My mom's life experiences, her wisdom and resilience, have shown me that she's navigated many of these paths already. And through her, I've learned that I will be okay too.

The response to *Duty Free* has been overwhelming. It struck a chord with millions, revealing that the hardships my mother faced were not unique but rather a widespread, yet underrepresented, reality. This feedback reinforced my commitment to tell these stories, highlighting the daily beauty and pain in caring for loved ones. After the film's success, we engaged in advocacy work, discussing age inclusivity with companies, lobbying with Congress for laws to protect older Americans, and speaking at retirement homes. These experiences led me to my next project on multigenerational housing, exploring how families manage and benefit from living together across generations.

Living with my mother for three years, post-film, taught me that intergenerational relationships, while enriching, are not without their hurdles. This realization is vital for my current projects, including a podcast, where I aim to delve deeper into these intricate and profound intergenerational dynamics. Through my work, I've come to understand the importance of preparing for and embracing the responsibilities of caring for aging family members. It's a time filled with hard conversations, growth, and ultimately, a deeper connection and understanding of life itself. My mission is to continue exploring and sharing these stories, to inspire others to embrace intergenerational connections and the richness they bring to our lives.

It's important to acknowledge and embrace these complexities as part of the journey. I've noticed we often shy away from acknowledging its complexities. Many of us in this field tend to gloss over the challenges because there's a pervasive fear of the 'hard stuff' in these relationships. There's a sense that we must portray these connections as perfect and wholly positive, possibly because mainstream media doesn't frequently showcase the nuanced narratives of intergenerational care and bonding. We might be worried that if we highlight the difficulties, people might be less inclined to value these connections, especially when they're not easy.

The reality, however, is that while intergenerational relationships can be challenging, navigating misunderstandings or disconnects helps us reach the truly meaningful moments. Facing these challenges is essential; it's part of what it means to be alive and to connect with others at a deeper level. Intergenerational connection isn't just about casual conversations or sharing past stories. It's about exploring who we are at our core, learning about ourselves through someone else's experiences. It's crucial to make these connections, even if it means engaging in difficult conversations. As we all age, we desire to be understood for who we are and how we've lived.

MICHAEL ROSSATO-BENNETT

Executive Director of the Alive Inside Foundation and Director, Writer, and Producer of the film Alive Inside

aliveinside.org

Alive Inside is a joyous cinematic exploration of music's capacity to reawaken our souls and uncover the deepest parts of our humanity.

"There's a profound magnetic connection between the young and the old, representing the two ends of our existence—those who are closest to beginning and those who are closest to the end."

Like many in our culture, I felt lost for a long time, without understanding why. As a child, I escaped into fantasy stories and imaginative worlds. I loved storytellers like Steven Spielberg who could take imagination and turn it into hope and solace for others. I wanted to be like that, but I lacked the confidence to realize my dream. I ventured into filmmaking, creating various artistic, corporate, and comedy films, just trying to hone my skills. Eventually, I became a father and had to prioritize providing for my family. I became a 'hired gun' filmmaker. I hadn't made my dream come true. I hadn't told a story that gave people sustenance and changed lives.

And then one day I got a job which was to follow this guy around for a day. Dan Cohen, who later created the Music & Memory program, had this idea that when people went to nursing homes, they left all their music at home. That made him sad. Using iPods and headphones, he wanted to give them the music they had loved and left behind. We went to a nursing home and gave music to a 94-year-old man with dementia named Henry. As I filmed him, we placed headphones over his ears. He appeared utterly lost, but as he listened to the gospel and Cab Calloway songs from his youth, something remarkable happened.

The music woke up some deep part of his brain and he started speaking pure poetry—pure human beauty erupted out of him. After sitting in a corner for ten freaking years, *TEN years*, slumped over in a corner, this man was now totally alive. Witnessing Henry's transformation was like watching Lazarus wake from the dead. He seemed to have gone from lifelessness to full vitality. This man had spent a decade, a full ten years, in silence and solitude. The awakening was profound. What struck me most was the way the music not only transformed Henry but seemed to ripple into everyone in the room, even those far gone in dementia. It sent shivers down my spine, too. It was a revelation, a slap in the face that completely altered my perception of life and its possibilities. The experience made me realize I had shut down a part of myself, and I needed to rediscover my own inner life. How was it possible that a 94-year-old man with dementia was more alive than I was?

A few days later, I gathered all my music and retreated to my bedroom. I decided I would listen to my music and see if I could find some glimmer of the light that shone in Henry. Here I was, a man with two children and a loving wife, seemingly successful in the world, but deep down, I knew I was only half alive. It was a moment of realization, you know? A chance encounter with an older man made me embark on a life-changing journey. It made me think, "Hold on, I could do something incredible here." There are 1.5 million individuals in institutions and at home who are essentially warehoused, lost due to the way our culture operates. We're all so individualized and atomized that intergenerational connections are becoming rare. The sad truth is, in order to meet our societal obligations, we have to medicate and warehouse our elders—not always, of course, but that's the way it feels.

I thought, *what if I tell a story and inspire people to improve life for a million elders?* I didn't know if it was feasible, and I was trying to make it happen with limited resources, but I persevered. Then, a year in and quite by accident, a clip of Henry I'd sent to a woman appeared on Reddit after it was found on her laptop, by her son.

It went worldwide viral almost overnight. This was during the early days of the internet when 'viral' truly meant something special. There was no paid promotion; it spread because people loved it and shared it with everyone they cared about—authentic virality, you know? It was just a small part of the film, not intended to be shared, but it going viral revealed to me that I was not alone—the entire world needed awakening.

So, I made this film, *Alive Inside* and it ended up winning the Sundance Film Festival Audience Award for a U.S. Documentary, and then things got pretty wild. The film was showcased at 110 film festivals, and it gained a lot of attention. It played on Netflix and Amazon. In the film, you see Dan Cohen and I get music into thirty-two nursing homes. However, the release of the film expanded our reach significantly. Our dream was coming true, the dream of providing older adults with the music of their youth, and touching that deep, emotional, and physical part of the brain that remains alive until the very end of our lives, even for those with Alzheimer's.

It was an incredible journey, and I felt a tremendous sense of joy witnessing how people were moved by our efforts. I think many people realized they weren't as alive as this older man, Henry. He had grown up inside the music, been immersed in the beat of life, and that connection still pulsed through his body. Was he showing us something we had lost? Henry told me he had always dreamed of being a singer, but ended up a janitor. But, isn't it amazing? In the end, his voice touched millions and helped change the way the world sees dementia. That's incredible, isn't it?

Through the success of the film, the music idea expanded to around 10,000 nursing homes internationally. That was amazing, but I soon realized the institutions were not signing up for the same dream. The institutions saw the music as a low-cost demonstration that they were doing something, as a distraction, as a way to kick the can down the road for a few years. What they were really focused on was continuing to profit from drug sales and housing fees. It made me sad. The appearance of doing good trumped my awakening dream. Even worse, I noticed, that the initial enthusiasm for the music program faded. The majority of the music players ended up locked away in drawers in about half of the organizations that had signed up.

I called my friend Tony Fisher, who ran Healdsburg Senior Living in California, and I asked the question, "What if kids bring music to older adults?" Answering that question started by showing the film *Alive Inside* at the schools, guiding kids through dementia exercises, and then bringing the students to meet with older adults and find their music. We called it 'CommUniversity.' Initially, I thought what we were doing was bringing youthful energy to the elders, but it soon became apparent that the kids needed the experience just as much, if not more, than the older adults did.

Young people often live a somewhat empty existence, disconnected from the richness of life. There's a profound magnetic connection between the young and the old, representing the two ends of our existence—those who are closest to beginning and those who are closest to the end. Throughout our history, the older generation has borne the responsibility of passing down wisdom to the younger one. Everyone knows how grandparents are nicer to their grandchildren than they are to their own children. Watching this magic unfold in front of me, I felt like I had been given another bite at the apple, another opportunity to make a difference, to reduce a huge suffering.

I was excited about the potential of combining two seemingly broken institutions, healthcare and public education, and creating something truly transformative. In our culture, many American children are left with more devices and less deep interactions. What we were doing was insane. We were asking them to change the life of an adult! This is a rare opportunity in our world and has profound implications. I started documenting everything that was unfolding in front of me. Three months in, COVID-19 struck and everything we'd been working on came to a grinding halt. Four years of work got dismantled overnight. Now, we all understood what it felt like to be disconnected and locked away!

I experienced my own 'dark night of the soul' during the pandemic. The dream I had spent my entire life building fell apart, breaking my heart. It became clear that it was meant to fall apart for a reason. I wasn't truly aligned with my authentic self. I had been living in survival mode my whole life. Sadly, as I traveled through this, I realized there are many people who live in this disconnected state. What I discovered on my journey is there are ways for human beings to reconnect with their true selves, and music and empathy are the truest pathways to that reconnection.

Now, wiser, I've reunited my team and we're relaunching the CommUniversity program, and resuming the documentary. We have ten institutions lined up, and if all goes well, in a year or two we'll have 1,000 elder communities partnering with 10,000 public schools. My goal is not just to create a program for nursing homes and schools but to help people of all ages live authentically. The aim is to support individuals on their journey back to their vibrant, essential core as human beings, even in the brief span of our mortal lives.

Music is our ally. It holds ancient wisdom that emerges from the heartbeat of our mother. It represents the tribal rhythms that resonate within us, waiting to be unleashed. Luckily, this profound and essential song lies dormant in each of us, and is very strong in the young and the old. This song needs to be reawakened, and it can be. By connecting the young and old through music and empathy, we can transform all our lives and rediscover the gifts of our shared and innate capacity to perceive and pursue beauty.

JON ADAM ROSS

Executive Director and Co-Founding Artist
Inheritance Theater Project

inheritancetheater.org

Connecting intergenerational, interfaith and intersectional communities to transcend divisions through a participatory playmaking process.

"We're building relationships across divides through a participatory playmaking process that uses cultural touchstones to activate conversations on the cultural, socio-economic, religious, and racial legacies of communities."

Ever since I was a kid, I wanted to live a life in the theater. I thought I had to be one of the Genes (Hackman, Wilder, Kelly). But I was fortunate enough to have incredible teachers, especially at the New York University (NYU) Tisch's Experimental Theatre Wing. They taught me that theater doesn't just have to be made for audiences, it can be made *with community.* I learned clowning, miming, Afro-Haitian tribal dance, street theater, and applied theater for social change. I was hooked on all the different ways stories can be told to serve communities.

I was also reared with a sense of civic responsibility. I grew up in Memphis, TN, with a grandmother who passed on a legacy of activism. Selma Lewis, white and Jewish, became a historian focused on documenting the Civil Rights Movement in real time. Her work interviewing the wives of sanitation workers in Memphis helped bring attention to the absurd poverty wages that galvanized the strike in 1968. Grandma Selma's house was just down the street from my high school, and I would walk there after school for a snack and a visit in between my last class and whenever rehearsal would start for whichever play I was working on. My grandmother went back to get her Ph.D. in history in the 1970s after raising her three kids and then became a history professor at a local university. She became a lay leader for social service organizations and helped start a national nonprofit called Facing History and Ourselves. Being attuned to, and actively engaging in social justice, was ingrained in me from an early age. One thing I learned from my Grandma Selma is that the process is as important as the end result. And that plays a big role in how I do the work I do today.

Participatory playmaking can lower the barrier of entry to relationships, and those relationships can and will strengthen communities. Doing our work intergenerationally allows for perspectives of the past, the present, and the future to inform the art that gets made. Communities are inherently intergenerational. And our work as artists facilitating this open process must engage as many constituent stakeholders as possible. That means intergenerational work is a necessary core to everything we do. I've spent the past twenty years looking for opportunities to build community through the process of storytelling, not just the performance at the end. This is reflected in our approach at the Inheritance Theater Project (ITP).

In Minneapolis, we facilitated a movement and storytelling workshop in partnership with a local dance company for older adults and preschoolers. The material generated by older adults and preschoolers contributed not only to our final product, but to a separate play devised and performed by high school students.

In Seattle, a visual arts project emerged parallel to our playmaking process, where women of all ages decorated the lenses of costume eyeglasses to express their own impressions of sister relationships, under the artistic direction of local visual artist sooze bloom deLeon grossman.

At the height of early COVID-19, we facilitated an online series of 'salons' where artists would bring in work responding to a shared prompt and get input and response from other artists in the ITP community. The ages of participating artists ranged from early twenties to late seventies. And it was exciting to see how artists jumped in to connect with each other's work. Eventually, some intergenerational collaborations ensued with really exciting results.

Most excitingly, in 2022-2023 we facilitated a project in Memphis, with support from the National Endowment for the Arts and in partnership with the Smithsonian's National Civil Rights Museum at the Lorraine Motel, to commemorate the 55th anniversary of Dr. Martin Luther King's assassination. For that project, we partnered with Creative Aging of the Mid-South to connect with elders from residential centers in different zip codes around Memphis, bringing them together to generate and shape material for the play. We also worked with Facing History and Ourselves (thanks, Grandma Selma!), to work with private and public school students from different areas of town as well. Eventually, we were able to bring the older adults and students together for a capstone performance of the finished play that they had all helped to create, followed by a two-hour pizza lunch where three students and three elders sat at each table, debriefing the process and the play. That was a really special day for our entire team, and for the community. Out of our efforts, Facing History and Creative Aging (organizations that have co-existed in the community for a long time without collaborating) are now in relationship and talking collaboration beyond our time on the ground in Memphis.

It's been thrilling to do this work around the country. Since its founding in 2015, the Inheritance Theater Project has employed over 240 artists and partnered with over 400 community organizations to engage over 11,000 people in 16 cities around the United States. An extra bit of excitement is that a PBS short documentary about our work won an Emmy award in 2023, and a full length PBS documentary will air in 2024, with even another one of our projects slated to be the subject of a new documentary later next year. The storytelling around the impact of this work inspires us to keep moving forward to bridge divides in more communities here in the States and around the world (we did our first international project in Rwanda in 2023, with more global projects set to come in the near future). Silos exist. Art can help.

JAKE ROTHSTEIN

Founder & CEO of Upside, Co-Founder of Papa

joinupside.com

Building the largest senior living community in the world—without laying a single brick.

papa.com

Pairing older adults and families with Papa Pals for companionship and assistance with everyday tasks.

"The value of intergenerational connections, a core lesson from both Papa and Upside, is immense. These connections combat loneliness and foster a sense of purpose across generations."

My path in this longevity industry is deeply personal, shaped by my experiences with my grandparents. It began with my grandfather's Alzheimer's diagnosis, a challenging time for my grandmother, who at 82, became his primary caregiver. She managed this for about four or five years, largely keeping the extent of her efforts from the family.

My grandmother would call me a few times a week to ask if I would sit with my grandfather for a few hours so that she could get some relief from her caregiving duties. She was still healthy and active with a network of friends, and I was able to provide a respite from her responsibilities, allowing her brief escapes to meet friends.

Over time, that got cumbersome and challenging. I remember one day sitting at the kitchen table with my grandfather, who, at that point, knew I was familiar, but he didn't really know who I was. I decided to contact several home-care agencies, seeking someone to simply be with him at short notice. He needed someone that could just sit with him at a moment's notice to make sure he was safe, while my grandmother got a little break. I called five places, and all five of them were the same. Despite my grandmother managing his primary care, the agencies insisted on minimum hours and a set schedule. That was just not going to work for my grandmother. We needed something more flexible.

It was 2015, a time when technology was revolutionizing services with the gig economy. Everyone was talking about using technology to make things more efficient. Seeing a gap in the caregiving world, I partnered with my cousin Andrew Parker, who had telemedicine experience and founded the company Papa, named after what we called our grandfather. It was a simple yet revolutionary idea: use the new gig economy model to pair the twenty million college students that were looking for flexible work with older adults that needed some extra assistance and companionship.

Papa was initially a direct-to-consumer service, and it has now evolved into a significant player in the healthcare sector. To date, Papa has completed over two million visits nationwide, primarily collaborating with health insurance companies. The inception of this company put me on a trajectory of working in this longevity space. It wasn't just a business venture; it was a heartfelt response to a gap I experienced in my own family.

As Papa grew, addressing this gap in care, my grandmother's situation also evolved, presenting new challenges. My grandmother just physically couldn't take care of my grandfather anymore and had to move him into a traditional senior living community. At 87 years old, my grandmother was now on her own for the first time in her adult life. She had never handled financial matters or house maintenance before, and this was all new territory for her. The urgency of the situation became apparent when we discovered that she was depleting her savings rapidly due to the $11,000 monthly expense of my grandfather's memory care facility.

Our family recognized that we needed to take action. We had to sell the house, as she couldn't navigate the stairs and had recently undergone knee replacement surgery. Despite her initial reluctance, we encouraged her to make this difficult decision. We found her a rental apartment in the same neighborhood, close to her doctors, friends, and grandchildren. This move significantly improved her quality of life. She no longer had the constant worry of running out of money, thanks to the equity from the house. The apartment was well within her financial means, allowing her to live out the rest of her life in relative health and happiness, free from the financial and physical burden of a house she could no longer afford or maintain.

This experience served as the inspiration for UpsideHōM (now 'Upside'). Traditional senior living facilities cater to only 10% of older adults, leaving the remaining 90% grappling with the same challenges my grandmother faced. They are left to figure out how to manage their homes, downsize, and make important life decisions with limited attractive alternatives. Some may move in with their children or settle in a retirement community they can't truly afford, while others may opt for one-bedroom apartments in older neighborhoods, often feeling isolated from society as they age.

Upside was conceived to address these issues, offering a new kind of senior living experience that maintains independence and promotes community engagement. We set out to build the biggest senior living community in the world, without laying a single brick, by partnering with existing apartment communities, ensuring they are age appropriate and accessible, and provide a range of services tailored to the needs of older adults.

The value of intergenerational connections, a core lesson from both Papa and Upside, is immense. These connections combat loneliness and foster a sense of purpose across generations. Upside extends this philosophy, integrating older adults into diverse, multi-generational communities, where the wisdom of age and the vibrancy of youth can coexist and benefit each other.

My work in intergenerational services is a blend of personal mission and professional endeavor. It's about transforming the challenges faced by my own family into opportunities for better, more connected ways of living for all generations. It's not just providing services; it's about creating communities where generations can learn from and support each other, enhancing everyone's quality of life.

SAMUEL RUBIN

Co-Founder and Impact Officer
Hollywood Climate Summit

hollywoodclimatesummit.com

Creating a community space for thousands of cross-sector entertainment and media professionals to take action on climate.

"Every year, we collaborate with our grassroots and movement partners to encourage our community to take climate action in the ways that we each uniquely can."

My passion for intergenerational advocacy and research developed as a result of cultivating personal experiences and forming meaningful relationships with individuals across diverse age groups. Growing up, my grandparents played a significant role in my life. I remember how my friends used to think my grandfather was the coolest person ever because he could do all these incredible magic tricks. He was even a member of the Magic Castle in Los Angeles, an exclusive private club for magic enthusiasts, and I cherished the times he took me along. He taught me that anyone could be a superhero—focused and precise, but also creative and imaginative.

This early exposure to intergenerational knowledge made me realize the importance of bridging generations and exchanging life experiences. My grandparents always rooted for me unconditionally and were very supportive of my creative endeavors. They attended my theater plays, applauded the loudest at my screenings, and generously allowed me to shoot my student films at their own house (a gesture only those who truly care would make).

Seeing and treating my grandparents as if they were friends provided me with a safe space that allowed me to express my authentic self without repercussions. One of our most cherished activities was watching our favorite TV shows together. I always felt so lucky that we had similar tastes in entertainment, and I appreciated them supporting the industry that I am also a part of. For these and so many more reasons, I always felt comfortable discussing anything with them, even things like drugs or relationships.

I've consistently challenged societal norms. When I started dating my first boyfriend, forty-seven years older than me, they didn't judge or object; instead, they embraced it wholeheartedly. Indeed, we went all together for a dinner date just about two weeks after we started dating. After we broke up, they invited him to my grandfather's 80th birthday party without even telling me beforehand. I guess the opposite of them not accepting him was to become best friends.

If breaking all these conventional norms taught me something, it is that intergenerational connections (of almost any kind) offer numerous benefits. First, they nurture diversity and the intersectionality of thought, fostering innovative and creative solutions. Different generations bring unique perspectives and insights to the table, enriching the collective knowledge. Additionally, intergenerational work breaks down barriers and fosters empathy and understanding between people of all ages. It allows us to collaborate and create positive change together, breaking away from the competition that might arise in same-age settings. These connections are vital for building a resilient and cohesive society.

I have embedded these values and principles into the projects I've been involved in and co-founded, such as the Hollywood Climate Summit or the groundbreaking Entertainment and Culture Pavilion held at COP 28 (the United Nations Climate Conference). As a social impact strategist and content producer, I focus on leveraging the media to drive positive change in environmental justice and human rights. Spaces like the Summit or the Pavilion aim to communicate the nature of the entertainment and climate ecosystem, bringing together diverse partners to collaborate, share resources, and create sustainable change. We emphasize networking, intergenerational mentorship, and supporting young entertainment activists by providing opportunities to pitch their projects to industry executives.

Through these intergenerational efforts, I have witnessed tangible improvements in both the entertainment and climate sectors. The ecosystem of partnerships has grown, leading to more collaboration and enhanced efforts in addressing climate issues. We've facilitated connections between different organizations and helped them find common ground to work together towards shared goals. By providing platforms for young activists to pitch their projects, we've seen increased funding and support for their initiatives, creating a tangible impact on climate-related issues.

I look forward to witnessing the ongoing growth of The Hollywood Summit Climate, and I am thrilled to embark on an even more ambitious project with the development of the Entertainment and Culture Pavilion at COP 28, situated within a Blue Zone. This endeavor amplifies the relevance and urgency of intergenerational dialogues and dynamics. As we nurture intergenerational relationships and foster connections between different age groups, we create a more inclusive and resilient community. I am thrilled to contribute to the creation and fortification of community spaces for collective learning, networking, and collaboration. This ensures that we can effectively and creatively tackle climate challenges together.

PHILOMENA MORRISSEY SATRE

Director of Diversity and Inclusion and Strategic Partnerships, Land-O-Lakes

landolakes.com

For the love of dairy and our farmer-owners.

"Creating a workplace where everyone feels welcomed, heard and comfortable bringing their authentic self to work every day."

The seed for my generational work was planted years ago. My mom is an immigrant from Ireland and came to the United States at age 16 and is from a family of twelve kids. I had never met my Irish grandparents, nor my relatives who had not traveled to the United States. After college, I backpacked Europe with a friend. I had an opportunity to spend two weeks with my grandparents and learn our family history and better understand who I was. My grandparents were farmers, experienced many challenges, and yet maintained a spirit of generosity and positivity. That was one of my sparks.

I previously served for ten years on the board of a nonprofit called SHIFT. The focus of the nonprofit was serving people in midlife. SHIFT was a community hub for mid-lifers as they navigated work-life transitions, connecting them to resources, organizations and individuals that guided members to lives of purpose and impact. I learned so much about the challenges that people in midlife face at work and home, and that experience energized me to have a focus on aging in my workplace. In my current role leading Diversity-Equity-Inclusion (DEI) at Land O Lakes, we have eleven Employee Resource Groups (ERG).

Our ERG at Land O Lakes are employee-led with senior level executive sponsors. These groups work to help create a workplace where everyone feels welcomed, heard and comfortable bringing their authentic self to work every day. Two of these groups are focused on intergenerational connections. We have a Young Professionals ERG and an Aging Successfully ERG. They operate independently, and also co-sponsor events throughout the year. They host educational forums, volunteer in the community, support our efforts to recruit talent to Land O Lakes. This year, our Aging Successfully ERG, with the support of our organization, signed the AARP Pledge which supports the belief in equal opportunity for all workers. The pledge recognizes the value of experienced workers, and reinforces the importance of recruiting across diverse age groups and consideration for all applicants on an equal basis, regardless of age.

An intergenerational workforce offers a multitude of advantages. Among these, a standout benefit emerges when we consider the sharing of perspectives and experiences within and across teams. This exchange enriches our collective knowledge and skill set, providing a solid foundation for fostering innovation and facilitating creative problem-solving. The diverse life experiences we each bring to the table enhance our ability to address challenges and navigate conflicts effectively.

Another notable benefit is the impact of mentoring. At Land O Lakes, our Young Professionals Employee Resource Group (ERG) facilitates a reverse mentoring program. This initiative pairs experienced employees as mentees with young professionals as mentors. Each month, the program delves into various focus areas, ranging from Work-Life-Wellbeing to Technology and Career Development Strategies. Having personally engaged in this program for the past three years, I've had the privilege of learning invaluable insights from my mentors. This experience has deepened my understanding of the daily experiences of colleagues at the early stages of their careers.

Intergenerational connection fosters a deeper understanding among our employees. While there are numerous commonalities that bind us together, each generation also brings its unique strengths and perspectives. Embracing this diversity in understanding prevents us from falling into the trap of making judgments or relying on stereotypes, and it ensures that we appreciate the individuality of each person. This element is essential in building a culture where everyone feels valued, whether they are embarking on their career journey or reaching the pinnacle of their profession.

DERENDA SCHUBERT

Executive Director, Bridge Meadows

bridgemeadows.org

Using the power of community to help children heal from the trauma of foster care by offering high-quality affordable housing, therapeutic programs, and intergenerational support with elders as mentors, friends, and caregivers, forming a safety net of care and interdependence.

"We are knitting back the social fabric that isolation and economic struggles have torn apart, reminding everyone that they matter, regardless of their age."

My journey into intergenerational work was deeply personal. It all began with my family's story. My mother struggled with mental health conditions, which created challenging circumstances for our family. However, we were fortunate to have my grandmother and aunties step in and create a beautiful safety net around us. They ensured we had food, clothes, made it to school, and celebrated our achievements. This intergenerational support was a part of our Polish and European cultural heritage where interconnectedness among family members was the norm.

As I grew older, I began to appreciate the profound impact of this safety net. It wasn't just about practical help; it was about the emotional and social support we received. This realization led me to pursue a career as a child psychologist, specializing in working with children in foster care. I witnessed the absence of such support networks in many families. They were missing the vital safety net that could catch them when they fell, be it in moments of crisis or simply in the day-to-day challenges of life.

As my career evolved, I led a mental health agency. I noticed a recurring issue; clients would leave our care with fragile connections and limited support systems. It was a stark contrast to the security and support I had experienced during my childhood. That's when I was introduced to Hope Meadows, a pioneering intergenerational community in rural Illinois, where families adopting foster children live alongside older adults in a mutually supportive environment. The transformative power of human connection, and the potential for healing and growth in unconventional family structures, resonated with me.

This became the germ of the idea for Bridge Meadows, founded in 2005 in Portland, Oregon. Using the Hope Meadows model, we replicated affordable intergenerational communities, incorporating deliberate, trauma-informed architectural designs that facilitate healing within a communal setting. I realized this model held the key to addressing the pressing need for more sustainable and robust support systems. It was only later that I connected the dots between my personal experiences and my professional path. My family had been my safety net and I wanted to create something similar for others. Without their loving care, I wouldn't be where I am today.

The value of intergenerational connections is immeasurable. At Bridge Meadows, we've seen firsthand how all generations benefit from one another. Children gain not only practical support but also wisdom and guidance from their elder counterparts. Elders find renewed purpose in their lives, shedding feelings of invisibility and social isolation. They have a reason to wake up every morning and lead meaningful lives. This intergenerational exchange reduces ageism, a pervasive issue in our society, and fosters a sense of belonging.

Our children at Bridge Meadows develop strong foundations outside of their biological families. They have a network of people who care about them, celebrate their achievements, and provide guidance. Elders serve as confidants, offering valuable life lessons. Our children feel safe, stable, and seen, which is crucial for their development.

Bridge Meadows conducts assessments of resiliency to evaluate the youth's capacity to navigate resources and rebound from challenging situations. Impressively, all youth within the community have consistent access to sufficient daily meals, and they exhibit a high level of resilience. Additionally, a significant majority of these young individuals receive essential healthcare with 77% visiting a dentist for preventive care and 88% attending non-emergency, preventive well-child checkups, surpassing the rates seen among their peers in foster care.

Parents within the Bridge Meadows community also demonstrate resilience with 77% feeling confident in their coping abilities during crises. Furthermore, an equal proportion of parents report having access to social support from friends, family, and neighbors. These parents also highlight access to tangible goods and services that aid them in managing stress, especially in times of intensified need.

Elders in the community also thrive within this intergenerational environment. They boast an average flourishing score of 92%, indicating a strong sense of well-being and fulfillment in their lives. A substantial 89% of elders find support from their social networks, and 87% express that they lead meaningful lives, actively contributing to their happiness and well-being. These statistics illustrate the positive impact of the Bridge Meadows model on individuals across generations.

During the pandemic, a beautiful example of intergenerational connection emerged. One of our young residents expressed concern for the well-being of our elder residents. This act of caring transcended age barriers and exemplified the power of reducing ageism. It revealed how our young residents perceived their elders with humanity, recognizing them as individuals beyond the mere label of being in foster care.

Bridge Meadows is not just about housing; it's about creating and inspiring intergenerational communities. Families who have experienced foster care, along with elders from across the country, come together to form a supportive network. Our staff plays a pivotal role in knitting these communities together, ensuring everyone's needs are met and conflicts are resolved.

Bridge Meadows addresses the social determinants of health by providing stable housing, fostering economic development, and creating a strong sense of community. It's a model that brings different generations together, breaking down silos and illuminating what's possible when systems and people collaborate. We are knitting back the social fabric that isolation and economic struggles have torn apart, reminding everyone that they matter, regardless of their age.

BARBARA GREENSPAN SHAIMAN

Author, Live Your Legacy Now! Ten Simple Steps to Find Your Passion and Change the World, Founder and President, Champions of Caring and Embrace Your Legacy Now

championsofcaring.org

Inspiring, empowering, and activating changemakers of all ages and backgrounds to create social change.

"If you empower people of all ages to make social change, miracles can happen."

My mother used to compulsively brush her teeth, five or six times a day. My family was always late because at the last minute she would say, "Oh, my God, I have to go brush my teeth." Frustrated and impatient, we would ask her why she kept us waiting, but she never explained it.

Then, in 1988, my mother decided that my father, brother, and I should accompany her to Auschwitz where she had been incarcerated at the age of 19. My brother, the physician, thought this was a bad idea, that it would be too traumatic for my mother because she'd lost 65 relatives during World War II. But my mother insisted we go, and we arrived at the gates of Auschwitz accompanied by 40 of her Holocaust survivor friends and their children.

Standing anxiously at the gates under the sign that read, 'Arbeit Macht Frei' ('work will set you free'), my mother turned to me and said, "I was 19 years old. I had lost everyone and everything. I snuck a toothbrush into my dress; it was the last vestige of my humanity. I didn't have clean water while I was in the Lodz ghetto, let alone toothpaste. But just the feel of the bristles on my teeth made me feel human." Then she grasped my hand. "They took it away from me when I got to Auschwitz," she said.

I had such a visceral reaction to this story that I felt myself choking and I said, "Mom, I'm going to get some fresh air. I'll meet you back in the museum in a moment." And I broke down.

Once, outside, I saw these teenage German boys who were clowning around. I thought, "Who can behave this way at a killing place like Auschwitz?" I was born in Germany after the war, and German was my first language, so I walked over and asked them, "Do you know where you are? Don't you have respect? How can you act this way?" They started laughing even harder.

Right then, I had an epiphany, an insight. I decided that when I returned to Philadelphia, I wasn't going back to the national executive search firm I founded that recruited doctors. I wanted to work with young people to teach them about caring, kindness, and empathy. I wanted to empower them to make their voices heard about inhumanity and social injustice. And most of all, I aspired to help them develop the skill sets needed to become social entrepreneurs and address societal issues that resonated with them. My mother always encouraged me to, "Dream BIG. Dream in Technicolor." So that's what I decided to do.

Champions of Caring is the organization that I founded in 1995 in Philadelphia, Pennsylvania in response to that aspiration. My vision for this organization was to promote active participation and social change in response to the racism, religious and cultural intolerance, violence, homophobia, and poverty that I saw in our neighborhoods and our world. We assembled a team of educators to offer community and school-based programs that engaged people of all backgrounds, races, genders, and socioeconomic standing.

In light of the prevalent issues such as hatred, violence, and poverty that we observe in our society today, we believe it's essential for Champions of Caring to now evolve into a global movement. Our aim is to motivate individuals from all age groups and backgrounds to step up as changemakers. While our focus since 1995 has primarily been on schools and classrooms, we're now expanding our horizons. We aim to equip people from diverse backgrounds and age groups with the tools to work together in fostering social change while emphasizing intergenerational collaboration. Our website also includes tools and resources for individuals who are interested in starting their own social impact project.

My previous experience working with Title I (low income) students in the 1970s helped prepare me in this new venture. The youth were in trouble with the law, failing school, and in many cases didn't have significant role models. My role models were my mother, father, and grandmother, all Holocaust survivors. The resilience and life lessons that they taught me highlighted the importance of intergenerational bonding. The support and understanding from people who've experienced both extreme hardship and great joy propelled me to become the most impactful I could be. It was a gift they'd given me that I now wanted to pass on to my students.

I realized that when you put people together that need each other, miracles can happen. The youth didn't have supportive adults in their lives and many older adults at the local senior center were lonely, so

I paired them together. For many of these teens, this action resulted in less truancy, more engagement in school, improved grades, reduced incidents of misbehavior, and most important, the creation of meaningful and caring relationships.

Later in my career, I created a program where students from a Title One program at Kensington High School in Philadelphia met and shared their individual stories with Holocaust survivors. Despite their difficult life circumstances, these teens were greatly inspired by the stories of these survivors. Likewise, the survivors experienced joy in connecting with the teens. And although this event occurred fifteen years ago, several of those students (now in their thirties), recently told me that when they met the Holocaust survivors, it became the most significant learning experience of their entire high school career.

Clearly, there were several motivating factors and positive reasons that led me to start Champions of Caring. When we worked on social justice projects, the students operated in small committees with community experts that we recruited to help. These experts taught the students grant writing, public speaking, public relations and organizational skills. The students bonded with these experts, while the professionals acquired knowledge about these young people's thoughts, ideas, and goals. Because both groups gained tremendously from these experiences, it has solidified my belief that bringing different generations together creates an environment for success and growth.

Core elements of the program incorporate service and social impact, lessons of the Holocaust and all forms of genocide, and intergenerational collaboration and action. We have worked with 10,000 young people, from the greater Philadelphia region, who have given over a million hours of service locally, nationally, and globally to address homelessness, hunger, literacy, and other issues that their passion has led them to tackle.

A longitudinal study on the impact of our program was recently conducted by Dr. Kimberly Goyette, Chair of the Sociology Department at Temple University, who provided essential data on the positive outcomes of our intergenerational program. The positive outcomes include teaching students the skills of project organization, planning, and follow through; public speaking; using history to promote enlightened ideas; learning to work with diverse groups of people; and growing into leadership. Intriguingly, when students who participated in the program during the 1990s were interviewed decades later in their thirties and forties, a recurring sentiment emerged. These individuals profoundly valued the experience of meeting and collaborating with peers from various backgrounds. Many noted that during their youth, there weren't many platforms facilitating such diverse interactions. Our program, even in the 1990s, was pioneering in bringing these diverse student groups together, providing them an unparalleled platform for mutual understanding and collaboration.

Currently, we are producing a Champions of Caring documentary about teens from Philadelphia, now in their thirties and forties, who created their own projects for social change. We explore how the ventures impacted the lives of these ambassadors and we spotlight how they continue to give service, locally, nationally, or globally. We also ask, "Are they teaching their children, nieces, and nephews these same values of empathy, caring, and kindness?"

By sharing these stories of social justice work, we can showcase the achievements of the participants and our program. We hope to garner support to provide the necessary tools to inspire and empower a movement of intergenerational changemakers. We will also encourage future leaders of all ages to create campaigns that strengthen their communities around the world.

If you empower people of all ages to create social change, miracles can happen. Let's come together and create a better, kinder world for us and for future generations. The time is now.

NIKKI SHULTS

Executive Director, LBFE Boston

lbfeboston.org

Facilitating lasting intergenerational friendships through weekly social, educational, creative, and technology programs.

"Our vision is to help build inclusive, intergenerational communities, connecting young and old alike in the spirit of friendship."

I was very close with my grandmother growing up. My family lived in a rural part of Connecticut, about as rural as you can get in Southern New England. My grandparents were farmers, and my grandmother, who became a widow at a young age, lived in the center of our family compound. My two uncles built houses on either side, and my mom's house was across the street, so my extended family resided in close proximity.

I was the youngest grandchild among the eight of us. Despite my grandmother's partial deafness, we shared a strong connection, often communicating nonverbally. We played cards a lot, and she taught me how to play poker as soon as I could count. She loved playing cards with real stakes, so we had little margarine tubs filled with pennies at her house that we kept in a drawer in her bedroom. We would frequently raid those tubs and gather around the table for a card game. Whenever my mom would be looking for me, inevitably she would find me at my grandmother's house.

I remember the moment that I decided that I wanted to work with older adults as a career. It was during my high school years. My grandmother and I were playing cards, and in the midst of shuffling the cards, she paused and looked at me and said, "You're my favorite pal." It struck me profoundly, a mix of sadness and warmth. I had only one living grandparent while growing up; the other three had sadly passed away at a young age. I felt a sense of missing out on their presence.

Unlike many people who aspire to become teachers or work with children from a young age, I didn't particularly get along with kids when I was younger. Instead, I had always cherished my interactions with older individuals whether it was my grandmother, great aunt, or great uncle. That moment, playing cards with my grandmother, and her comment, solidified my desire to work with older adults as a career choice.

I studied gerontology at university and earned my MBA in healthcare management. Upon completing school, I initially began my career in social work. While I have immense respect for case managers and social workers, I quickly realized that this path wasn't the right fit for me. I took a detour and joined the Peace Corps for a few years. Toward the end of my time there, I served as the volunteer coordinator.

When I started in my current role at Little Brothers, Friends of the Elderly (LBFE) it was in the role of a volunteer coordinator. It felt as if everything in my life had led me to that moment, and I've now been here ten years.

LBFE is an international organization with its origins dating back to 1946 in France. Our founder, Armand Marquiset, embarked on this journey as a response to the aftermath of World War ll and the passing of his great philanthropist aunt. Seeing that many young lives had been lost in the war, and realizing that translated into a lack of care for older adults, he made it his life's calling and mission.

In 1946, Les Petits Frères des Pauvres, literally translated as 'The Little Brothers of the Poor,' was founded in France. Armand Marquiset's dedication was particularly focused on assisting the most destitute elderly people, and he soon realized that the hardest thing for them to bear was the overwhelming loneliness and isolation they experienced. This revelation became the guiding principle of his life's work.

The International Federation was established in 1979 and brings together organizations located in ten countries around the world. In the United States, LBFE has regional headquarters in Boston, Cincinnati, Chicago, New York, San Francisco and Upper Michigan. While their programs vary by location, each chapter is committed to establishing authentic and lasting friendships with isolated and lonely older people in their communities, inviting people of all ages and backgrounds to help combat this social epidemic and build a more inclusive society.

In Boston, we do that through intergenerational programs. We have three core programs.

The first one is known as CitySites, where we collaborate closely with Boston College and Northeastern University, along with a few other institutions. In this program, university students participating in service-learning initiatives are brought into public and affordable senior housing communities. By doing this, we ensure that the programs are accessible to older residents without the need for transportation or overcoming other barriers. CitySites primarily focuses on fostering social connections. The activities are tailored based on the interests of both older and younger participants. This could involve games, conversation circles, memoir writing, arts projects, and more. The activities serve as a platform for friendships to blossom and create opportunities for older and younger individuals to interact, which can be a rare occurrence in many settings.

Our second program, Digital Dividends, was initiated in response to the digital divide exacerbated by the pandemic. We address digital equity by providing classes to groups of ten to fifteen older adults, also residing in public and affordable housing. Participants receive a free Chromebook that they can keep, along with a hotspot with unlimited data for the duration of the approximately three-month program. Students from local universities involved in service-learning programs play a crucial role in teaching older adults how to use these digital tools. This three-pronged approach aims to enhance digital literacy among older adults, ensuring they have the necessary skills and access to the internet.

Finally, our third program, Creative Connections, differs from the others, as it is not intergenerational. Instead, we invite local artists to conduct six to eight-week fine arts courses. These courses encompass various artistic expressions, including painting, mixed media, dance, and more.

Collectively, through these three programs, we strive to replicate the social engagement and educational opportunities available to older adults in market-rate housing, extending these benefits to individuals residing in housing with fewer resources.

It is widely acknowledged that the challenges of loneliness and isolation have been a longstanding concern for older adults, not only during the pandemic but even before it. This issue is particularly pronounced among the individuals we work with who often face linguistic barriers. Consequently, we have found our niche in collaborating with non-native English speakers, including many international students. Last year, we were able to offer programs in up to nine different languages.

Our intergenerational programs, in conjunction with working alongside international students, offer a unique opportunity for meaningful community engagement. One distinctive aspect of our program model is its ability to eliminate transportation and cost barriers, as all our programs are provided free of charge. This allows older adults to age in place while facilitating conversations with individuals from different generations.

By operating within senior housing communities, where neighbors are typically in the same age bracket, our programs introduce a refreshing dynamic. Older adults benefit not only from gaining digital literacy skills and improving their communication abilities but also from the relationships they develop with younger generations. The importance of social engagement, especially as we age, cannot be overstated. Research indicates that socially isolated individuals over a certain age have a 26% higher likelihood of developing dementia or memory loss at a younger age. Both Gen Z and older adults are seeking interaction, meaning, and a sense of purpose in their lives. However, numerous barriers, akin to the "Okay, boomer" stereotype, often stand in the way.

We have conducted studies of our programs collaborating with the Northeastern Public Evaluation Lab, affiliated with Northeastern University. Their involvement has allowed us to collect data over approximately five years. The metrics we focus on include assessing the sense of connection, frequency of loneliness, willingness to assist neighbors in need, and comfort in seeking help from neighbors. Additionally, we gauge attitudes toward different generations.

The findings from these studies consistently show that intergenerational programs have a positive impact on reducing feelings of loneliness and isolation for both older and younger participants. Individuals feel free to ask questions they might hesitate to pose to their loved ones, ultimately fostering a unique opportunity for mutual learning and growth. They foster better perceptions of different generations and enhance a sense of community and connection.

HELEN HIRSH SPENCE

CEO and Founder, Top Sixty Over Sixty

topsixtyoversixty.com

Advocating for age diversity, equity, and inclusion.

"The 50-plus population's diverse contributions to labor markets support jobs and create opportunities for all."

My journey into intergenerational work has been a lifelong one, shaped by my extensive career in education, spanning over 55 years. Throughout this time, I have always found myself immersed in environments where multiple generations naturally coexisted. Whether as a student or an educator, I spent most of my professional life in schools where generations intertwined seamlessly. Reflecting on my career, I realize that I was always surrounded by people of varying ages.

As a secondary school principal and as head of an all-girls' school, I had the privilege of working with students of all ages, from junior kindergarteners to high school seniors. My interactions weren't limited to students; I also engaged with parents, grandparents, trustees, directors, the community, and superintendents. My professional life had always been a multigenerational one, and I welcomed the exchanges I had with young people, particularly teenagers.

The enthusiasm and refreshing outlook on life that young people bring have always inspired me.

For instance, my granddaughter, who was four years old at the time, once told me she was digging for bugs because, "Oma, I have to practice becoming a vet." I marveled at how she interpreted the need to prepare for her 'then' chosen profession by finding bugs. It was such a different way of perceiving the world.

A high school student, Laura Batson, on returning from a three-month adventure in the Himalayas, encouraged me to consider trekking too. Her support and encouragement resulted in my expedition through Nepal during the Maoist insurrection. Saumya Krishna, also a high school student, introduced me to social impact investing, which led me to take courses in social entrepreneurship and the founding of my current social enterprise. These interactions with younger generations have been life-changing for me.

All these personal experiences reinforced my belief in the merits of intergenerational interactions. It's not just about older generations imparting wisdom; it's a two-way street. I cherish the opportunity to learn from younger people and gain fresh viewpoints. It's essential to see the world through different lenses, especially in a world that places great emphasis on innovation and creativity.

In today's rapidly changing world, staying current and adapting to evolving paradigms is crucial. This can best be achieved by fostering relationships across generations and embracing different perspectives. Intergenerational work allows us to share expertise, skills, responsibilities, workloads, knowledge, housing solutions and so much more. The benefits of these exchanges far outweigh any potential drawbacks.

Throughout history, humans have naturally lived in multigenerational households out of necessity. It's only in the last century that we've started segregating ages. We've witnessed a shift from agrarian to industrial societies, leading to age-segregated schooling and, more recently, the separation of older adults into retirement homes and communities. In my opinion, this trend is misguided and deprives us of the richness that intergenerational connections offer.

Today, we live in a world with up to six and seven generations coexisting simultaneously and five generations working together. I strongly believe in generativity—the idea that each of us should pay forward our accumulated knowledge and experience to benefit future generations. This can be done through formal and informal mentorship, but in today's world, mentorship needs to be reciprocal and mutual. The old model of the wise mentoring the uninitiated is passé. Young people today have different outlooks and skillsets to offer. We all need to embrace new information, have a growth mindset, and shift our thinking.

I founded Top Sixty Over Sixty because I saw a need to address the impact of ageism on all generations, with a particular emphasis on older adults. Through our various programs, training, and thought leadership we showcase inspirational older adults who serve as role models for people of all ages. We advocate for age diversity in the workplace, and we teach older adults to recognize their own internal age bias. We want to change the ageing narrative for both young and older adults.

Our intergenerational events consist of facilitated conversations under the banner, "We Need to Talk." These discussions advance rich exchanges on topics like aging, societal perspectives and expectations, family dynamics etc., and are open to people of all ages. They are incredibly enriching, providing valuable insights and fostering a deeper understanding of generational similarities and differences. We welcome a diverse group of participants, including young and older individuals from South Africa, Poland, Turkey, New Zealand, and various other corners of the world. I am passionate about continuing these dialogues and witnessing the growth of this intergenerational exchange.

Another dream of mine is to establish an Intergenerational Learning Hub, particularly in an entrepreneurial context. This would be a place where individuals of all ages come together to learn from and complement each other's knowledge and skills. It's a vision of a vibrant, innovative environment where intergenerational collaboration thrives.

My journey into intergenerational work has been one of continuous discovery and inspiration. I am committed to breaking down barriers, fostering mutual learning, and creating a world where all ages are valued and respected. Through Top Sixty Over Sixty and other initiatives, I hope to leave an age-positive legacy, one that truly embraces age diversity and one where ageism has been banished forever.

ENNY VAN ARKEL

Managing Director
Stichting Oud Geleerd Jong Gedaan:
Old Learned, Young Done

oudgeleerdjonggedaan.nl

Connecting students to older adults to provide an opportunity for intergenerational, lifelong learning.

"Our dream is big: a more positive view of older adults and greater inclusivity."

The image of older adults needs to become more realistic, more positive, and especially, more inclusive. In the media, you mainly read about languishing, filled with misguided stories about pathetic and lonely elderly people. The image that is portrayed is not exactly what we as humanity should aspire to. How is it possible that we have come to see older adults as a separate target group instead of people, but with more life experience? Generations have become so distant from each other that we no longer see the beauty, only the limitations. How is it possible that my first large-scale experience with older adults was through a summer job? Before that it did not even occur to me to work with and for them.

The answer, in my view, is simple: what we don't know, we fear.

In the summer of 2011, I crossed the threshold of a nursing home for the first time in my life. I was studying Child Development and Education at the University of Amsterdam and had haphazardly mailed my curriculum vitae (CV) to several organizations because I wanted to work full time during the holidays. Amsta, a large health care organization in Amsterdam, was the first to respond, and I started working as hostess on a ward for people with dementia. Until then, dementia was a concept that I sometimes read about in the newspaper. When I thought of the elderly, I thought of my own grandparents. After all, they were over seventy years old and *so very old.* With no clue of what to expect, I started this holiday job. I lost my heart to the residents, and after my holiday job, I completely changed my career path.

Every day, I found it an incredible honor and challenge to make the residents feel at ease in the last phase of their lives. I learned a great deal from the daily contact with 'my' residents and developed an incredible drive to contribute to increasing their happiness in life. They, in turn, taught me many lessons, such as the great ability to put things into perspective, to worry less about things that don't really matter, and to slow down and not constantly run around like a headless chicken.

For decades, there has been a lack of structural contact between different generations. People are becoming increasingly distant from each other. This has been reflected in young people's career choices: jobs without a focus on contact with older adults are seen as attractive by young students. These jobs are often low in salary, and this has everything to do with image.

In order to tackle this problem and make the image of our elders more positive, a good friend and colleague and I set up the Oud Geleerd Jong Gedaan Foundation (roughly translated 'Old Learned, Young Done') in 2014, in the nursing home Ilse Nieuwland.

The idea is simple: students develop and give lectures on their discipline to older adults. Everyone should feel welcome at these lectures: people in nursing homes, living independently, with or without dementia, with an academic education or never having been to school. Interaction between young and old is central to this because although the student 'lectures,' we guide them in how they can give the older adults a platform to share their knowledge, opinion, and experience.

Thanks to our initiative, the students visit places where they would not otherwise easily go: nursing homes, rehabilitation centers, and community centers. The mere fact that they come out of their own bubble and broaden their horizons in this way is enormously valuable, and has an impact on many different levels.

Last month, there was a man with dementia at one of the lectures who completely flourished because he was learning about artificial intelligence and knew a lot about it himself. The week before, a woman with aphasia had made a deep impression on a student because she was suddenly able to string several words together when it came to her passion for art history.

The feedback from students is that they are enormously surprised by the extent to which all our participants are eager to learn. In addition, they find it very pleasant to be of added value by sharing their knowledge, and they learn a lot from the interaction with older adults. Thanks to the contact with older people that they have gained through this voluntary work, several students have now changed their career paths and are focusing on the care sector for older people.

JANINE VANDERBURG

Co-Founder, Changing the Narrative

changingthenarrativeco.org

Changing the narrative: ending ageism together.

"Imagine a world without ageism—one where the strengths and contributions of people of all ages are honored and appreciated, with public policies in place to ensure that all of us can thrive at any age. That's our vision, and one increasingly shared by many across the world."

Growing up in a French-Canadian and Portuguese community in Massachusetts, I was surrounded by an intergenerational way of life. One set of grandparents lived upstairs and the other just down the street. Our family business, a hardware store started by my immigrant grandfather, was a gathering place not just for commerce, but for familial and community interaction across generations. My dad and my uncle worked there, and as a child, I began working there at the age of five. Our customers were often fathers and sons working on projects together. It was a place where multiple generations of customers and employees interacted daily. I assumed this was the way people everywhere lived. I thought this was the norm—that intergenerational connections were a fundamental part of life.

As I moved into my thirties and started a consulting company, I continued to experience the power of intergenerational connections. My consulting career was predominantly populated by women, and our teams naturally spanned multiple generations. The intergenerational dynamic extended into my volunteer work in grassroots political campaigns. People of varying ages rallied together, united by shared causes and candidates. It seemed natural to me that people from different age groups would come together to work toward common goals.

Back in 2006, I got involved with Encore.org (now CoGenerate.org), and I was introduced to Marc Freedman's ideas about CoGenerate. I had been working on projects for two foundations about how people age 55-plus were thinking about their next phase of life. I presented the results of my research after hearing a keynote presentation by Freedman and became hooked. Years later (2018), I read his book *How to Live Forever: The Enduring Power of Connecting the Generations* and it sparked an idea.

In 2018, I founded Changing the Narrative, with a mission to change the way people think, talk and act about aging and ageism. Through evidence-based approaches, strategic communications, and innovative public-facing campaigns, we are committed to motivating people to take action against ageism and create a more age-inclusive society.

I realized the concept of intergenerational connections needed more attention and advocacy. Around the same time, conversations with my daughters and my son-in-law about the 'entitled millennial' stereotype highlighted the ubiquity of ageism and sparked an idea. What if we structured conversations that not only facilitated intergenerational connections but also incorporated educational elements about ageism?

This led Changing the Narrative to launch a campaign specifically focused on intergenerational conversations about ageism, aiming to dismantle it by any evidence-based means necessary. Research shows that when we have constructive conversations with people of all ages, about age and aging, coupled with education, that is the most effective way to reduce ageist attitudes. With this inspiration, we announced a bold plan: to host 100 intergenerational conversations about ageism in just over a month. We developed an Intergenerational Toolkit, and the campaign dubbed 'On the Same Page' took off.

Despite the challenge of a Colorado snowstorm that forced us to pivot some conversations online, the campaign was a success. The feedback was overwhelmingly positive, with participants reporting changed attitudes and a heightened understanding of ageism. The conversations didn't just resonate; they echoed widely, reaching beyond our initial scope, prompting interest internationally. The key takeaway from this experience was clear—intergenerational connections and education were potent tools in the fight against ageism. What made this approach particularly powerful was its acknowledgment that ageism affects both older and younger individuals. It dismantled the barriers that often divided generations and encouraged open and honest dialogue.

The momentum we'd built was, of course, challenged by the events of 2020. We shifted to virtual formats and created a televised PBS series on crucial topics, including the role of the arts in advancing social justice, digital divides during COVID-19, health equity, and ageism. However, one important lesson I learned during this time was that virtual discussions, while valuable, may not be as effective as in-person interactions. The ability to see and connect with people directly enhances the depth of the experience, making it more impactful.

The Intergenerational Toolkit is designed with three primary objectives in mind. It aims to cultivate awareness by promoting a collective understanding of the detrimental effects of ageism, emphasizing that ageism affects individuals of all ages, not just older adults. Second, it inspires reflection by encouraging individuals to consider the origins of ageism and strategies to combat it, fostering introspection and critical thinking. Finally, the toolkit seeks to foster engagement, motivating people to participate in ongoing discussions about ageism and identify actionable steps to address this societal issue.

We recently revamped the Intergenerational Toolkit to reflect the evolving landscape of resources and learning materials. This updated toolkit now encompasses both in-person and virtual options, along with questions that align with current research on ageism. Our goal is to provide a practical resource that empowers individuals and organizations interested in fostering intergenerational connections to combat ageism. I've found that the most powerful conversations often stem from simple questions about learning from different generations and personal experiences with age stereotypes. These discussions foster understanding and solidarity without triggering a defensive 'us versus them' mentality.

In addition, we have woven intergenerational elements into many of our workshops, ranging from addressing the business case for older workers and intergenerational teams in the workplace to broader discussions on ending ageism together. This approach has resonated particularly well with employers facing talent pipeline challenges and those seeking to foster age-inclusive workplaces.

Changing the Narrative, as a national campaign under the umbrella of the NextFifty Initiative, remains steadfast in its mission to end ageism. Our aim is not merely to raise awareness about ageism but to ignite the spark that drives people to act against it. We firmly believe that fostering intergenerational connections and education is a powerful tool in achieving this goal. We are committed to advocating for a world where ageism is eradicated, and people of all ages thrive together, creating a richer, more inclusive society for everyone.

DR. ROBERT G. WINNINGHAM, PH.D.

Former Chair of the Behavioral Sciences Division
Interim Dean of the College of Liberal Arts and Sciences

Professor of Psychological Sciences and Gerontology
Provost and VP for Academic Affairs
Western Oregon University

wou.edu/gerontology

From cognitive stimulation to technology integration and music therapy, our endeavor has evolved to encompass various approaches aimed at improving the cognitive and emotional well-being of residents in assisted living communities and memory care settings.

"My exploration of intergenerational work has been driven by a deep passion for enhancing the lives of older adults."

I've had the privilege of serving as a Provost and Vice President for five years before returning to teaching. My background lies in neuroscience, with a specialization in cognitive psychology and memory. In graduate school, I began my work focusing on how older adults remember crime scenes and related subjects, particularly in the context of eyewitness memory. This research laid the foundation for my interest in working with older adults and improving their cognitive well-being.

When I joined the university as a tenure-track professor, we had students collecting data in assisted living communities, a concept that started right here in Oregon. One of the things we became aware of was that many of these residents weren't engaged in meaningful activities during the day, and so we introduced cognitive stimulation experiments into their programming.

It was remarkable how much the residents loved it. It became a highlight for them, and we quickly realized that we needed to expand in this direction. This expansion led to the development of cognitive stimulation and brain exercise classes, and we conducted some groundbreaking randomized controlled studies in this area. We observed that these activities not only stimulated cognitive functions but also had a positive impact on the mental well-being of the residents, even though our initial focus wasn't on mental health.

As our work continued, we ventured into other avenues. We wanted to provide not just cognitive stimulation, but also a sense of purpose and meaning for the residents. Our studies found that by incorporating extended icebreaker activities and creating a social context within the brain exercise programs, we were able to decrease depressive symptoms and loneliness among our participants. We also explored the potential of technology, such as iPads, to enhance learning opportunities and engagement. With the largest undergraduate Gerontology program in the Pacific Northwest, we decided to get a grant, purchase iPads, and embark on a learning journey together with our students. It was a rewarding project that allowed us to connect with residents of different abilities and enrich their lives.

One of the most remarkable experiences was our foray into music therapy. We were inspired by a study that showed a decrease in the use of psychotropic medication among individuals in memory care communities who participated in our music initiative. We used services like Spotify to provide music to residents, some of whom had advanced dementia. The results were astonishing. People who couldn't communicate found a way to express themselves through music, sometimes even breaking into dance. It was a testament to the power of music in improving the quality of life for older adults.

Another notable project that emerged from student community practicums was the creation of an intergenerational dinner program, known as '50 Plus.' This program currently brings together college students, younger people, and older adults at the largest certified senior center in Oregon. Participants sit at tables of 10 to 12 people and use conversation starters to guide engaging discussions. This initiative has yielded surprising results, and we're currently conducting research to better understand its impact.

In our Gerontology department, we emphasize the importance of understanding social ties and aging, as these relationships play a pivotal role in supporting older adults. We've also initiated projects that promote social engagement, such as partnering with a high school for a 24-hour music fundraiser in assisted living communities. This endeavor brought joy and excitement to the residents, demonstrating the positive impact of intergenerational interactions in combating loneliness and enriching the lives of older adults.

During this time, I've written several books on the subject of memory and older adulthood. My first book, *Train Your Brain,* was an attempt to make academic knowledge on memory accessible to a broader audience. It covers various aspects of memory in older adulthood, including the limitations of mnemonics and memory tricks, the importance of social support, and the complex relationship between nutrition, aging, and memory.

My second book, *Cranium*, takes a different approach. It functions more like a workbook and includes adapted neuropsychological tests, allowing individuals to establish a baseline for their cognitive abilities. It also provides guidance on activities that target specific areas of the brain.

In a nutshell, *Train Your Brain* offers insights into memory improvement, while Cranium serves as a practical workbook to assess and enhance cognitive functions.

In recent years, I've observed a shift away from age-segregated communities, which is a positive development. College campuses, for instance, are now exploring the use of unused housing to create accommodations for older adults. This change aligns with the growing awareness of the loneliness epidemic in the United States, as highlighted by the Surgeon General's Health Advisory. Loneliness has been linked to significant health risks, and addressing it is becoming increasingly crucial.

My exploration of intergenerational work has been driven by a deep passion for enhancing the lives of older adults. From cognitive stimulation to technology integration and music therapy, the work has evolved to encompass various approaches aimed at improving the cognitive and emotional well-being of residents in assisted living communities and memory care settings.

REFLECTIONS

As I sit down to write these last words, the sun is setting on a decade that has reshaped my understanding of life. Approaching this project in the dawn of my fifties and now standing on the cusp of sixty, *Lives Well Lived* has been a journey of profound personal transformation and a testament to the power of human resilience, purpose, and the enduring strength of human connection.

From the very beginning, with a camera in hand and a vision in my heart, I set out to capture the essence of what it means to live a life filled with purpose, positivity, and resilience. The stories of the forty older adults I interviewed for the film were not just interviews; they were lessons in living. Each story brought to light the invaluable lessons of perseverance, the critical need for supportive networks, and the power of hope that defies life's challenges.

I've shared how *Lives Well Lived* evolved into a larger movement—one aimed at bridging the gap between generations. Inspired, I delved into the world of intergenerational work, discovering individuals and organizations globally who are creatively reuniting the young and old. The interviews shared, firsthand, the innovative ways to connect young and old, proving that our society thrives when it embraces inclusivity rather than segregation by age. This intergenerational dialogue is not just beneficial; it's essential for creating a world where wisdom is shared freely, where support systems are boundless, and where every individual (regardless of age) feels valued and heard.

This journey changed me. It deepened my appreciation for the interconnectedness of our experiences and the collective wisdom that guides us through life's ebbs and flows. It reminded me that, regardless of our backgrounds, the essence of what it means to live a good life is universal. This realization is my gift from the extraordinary individuals whose stories have filled these pages, and it's a gift I am now honored to share with the world inspiring a ripple effect of positivity and connection.

Now, as I approach a new decade in my life, the journey feels far from over. It continues to unfold, touching more hearts and inspiring more minds with each passing day. I am eternally grateful for the opportunity to share this journey with you and hopeful for the impact it will continue to have on the world.

As we close this book together, I invite you, the reader, to reflect on the lessons woven throughout these pages. The journey of *Lives Well Lived* is a testament to the enduring spirit of humanity and the transformative power of listening to and learning from each other. I hope these stories inspire you to seek purpose, foster resilience, build supportive communities, and cherish the connections that cross generational lines.

ABOUT THE AUTHOR

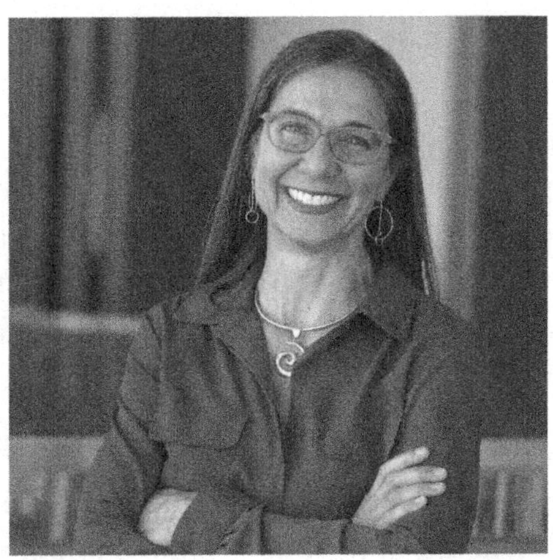

Originally embarking on a finance career, Sky Bergman's life took a turn during her final semester at the University of South Florida with a single photography class. Intrigued by the darkroom process, she pursued this newfound passion, earning an MFA in Photography from the University of California, Santa Barbara. Her photography found a place in prestigious collections like the Los Angeles County Museum of Art, the Brooklyn Museum, Seattle Art Museum, and the Bibliothèque Nationale de France. Her commercial work has appeared on book covers for Random House and Farrar, Straus & Giroux, Inc., and magazine spreads in Smithsonian, Arthur Frommer's Budget Travel, Reader's Digest, and Archaeology Odyssey.

After thirty years as a Professor of Photography and Video and former chair of the Art & Design Department at California Polytechnic State University, Sky is entering her "third act." Fueled by her passion for education and creativity, she's now focused on creating films and projects that bridge generational divides.

Following her successful directorial debut of the award-winning documentary, "Lives Well Lived," (currently airing on PBS), Sky directed "Forever Voters," exploring civic engagement between older adults and youth, and "Mochitsuki," which delves into the Japanese American experience as told through the tradition of making mochi to bring in the New Year.

Her latest project, "Prime Time Band," draws from her own experiences as a music enthusiast, telling the story of individuals united by their love for music. The film explores themes of purpose, community, and the timeless pursuit of passion, reflecting Sky's belief in the power of shared narratives to foster empathy and understanding across generations.

Her films are more than just stories; they are invitations to explore the depth of human connection across different stages of life. In 2022, Sky was named a CoGenerate Innovation Fellow, joining fourteen social entrepreneurs tackling major issues like racial inequality, climate change, and social isolation by uniting older and younger generations. She is an advocate for storytelling that bridges generations, enriching our collective understanding with every frame.

As an educator, artist, activist, and filmmaker, Sky Bergman remains intertwined with her mission to inspire, connect, and enlighten. Through her work, she continues to break down barriers of ageism, one story and one connection at a time. Her films celebrate the rich variety of life experiences and serve as a reminder that it's never too late to find your rhythm in life.

INSPIRE, CONNECT, AND LEARN

Enrich Your Community or Educational Institution with Sky Bergman's *"Lives Well Lived"* Screenings, Keynote Presentations, and Intergenerational Workshops

Discover the transformative power of storytelling and the wisdom of age through Sky Bergman's acclaimed documentary, *"Lives Well Lived."* This comprehensive program offers organizations, educational institutions, and communities an opportunity to inspire, connect, and engage audiences of all ages. Whether you're looking to host a thought-provoking film screening, invite Sky for a Q&A or presentation, or participate in enriching intergenerational workshops, Sky Bergman's offerings are tailored to foster understanding, appreciation, and collaboration across generations.

Host a Screening of "Lives Well Lived" with a Q&A Session

Overview: *"Lives Well Lived"* is a celebrated documentary that offers a heartwarming insight into the lives of people who have lived their decades with richness and authenticity. By hosting a screening of this film, organizations, educational institutions, and community groups have the unique opportunity to inspire and educate their audience about the beauty and wisdom of aging.

Features:

- **Engaging Q&A Session:** Following the screening, participants will have the chance to engage in a Q&A session with Sky Bergman, the filmmaker behind this powerful documentary. This provides a deeper understanding of the film's creation and the stories it shares.
- **Customizable Experience:** Depending on the audience, the Q&A session can be tailored to focus on specific themes such as resilience, joy, intergenerational connection, and the importance of storytelling in preserving history.

Keynote Presentations by Sky Bergman

Overview: Sky Bergman is available for keynote presentations where she shares her journey in creating "Lives Well Lived," the lessons learned from the lives she documented, and the critical importance of fostering intergenerational connections. Her talks are perfect for sparking inspiration and encouraging audiences to see the value in stories from older generations.

Features:

- **Inspirational Insights:** Sky brings to the stage a wealth of knowledge and insights from her interactions with individuals who have lived significant lives. Her stories inspire and challenge audiences to connect with older generations in meaningful ways.
- **Customizable for Various Audiences:** Whether for community groups, educational settings, or professional organizations, Sky tailors her presentation to resonate with the specific interests and needs of her audience.

Intergenerational Workshops & Programs

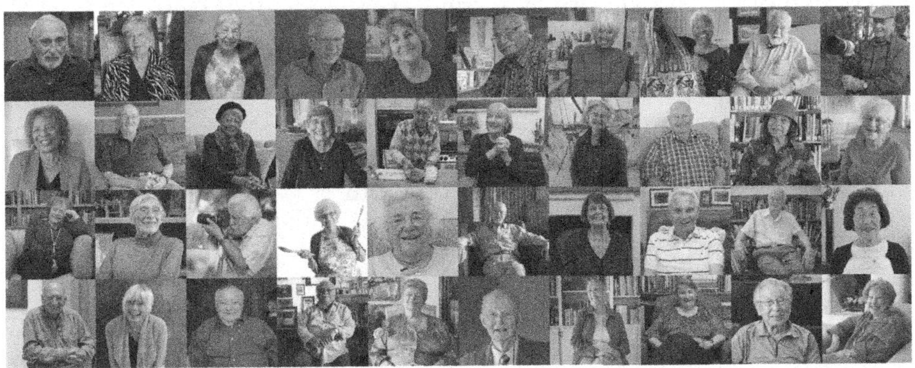

Overview: Recognizing the potential within a multigenerational workforce or community, Sky offers to customize educational experiences that explore and strengthen intergenerational connections. These workshops and programs are designed to foster understanding, collaboration, and mutual respect among participants of all ages.

Features:

- **Customized Educational Experience:** Every organization has unique dynamics and needs. Sky works closely with hosts to develop a program or workshop that best addresses the specific challenges and opportunities within their group.
- **Building Stronger Teams:** By emphasizing the value each generation brings to the table, these workshops help build more cohesive, understanding, and productive teams and communities.

Booking and Contact Information

To explore the possibility of hosting a screening of "*Lives Well Lived*," arranging for a keynote presentation by Sky Bergman, or discussing a customized workshop or program for your organization, please reach out through the following contact details:

Email: sky@skybergmanproductions.com

Invite Sky Bergman: Whether you are looking to inspire your community, educate your team, or celebrate the wisdom of older generations, Sky Bergman offers a range of opportunities to connect and learn. By hosting a screening, engaging Sky for a keynote, or participating in a workshop, you are taking a meaningful step towards bridging generational divides and enriching your organization's cultural and educational experience.

WAYS TO WATCH THE FILM

lives-well-lived.com/watch-the-film

AMAZON: bit.ly/LWLAmazon
iTUNES: apple.co/2YpODcI
PBS Passport: pbs.org/show/lives-well-lived/
KANOPY: kanopy.com/en/product/12391561
DVD: shop.pbs.org/WD7182DV.html

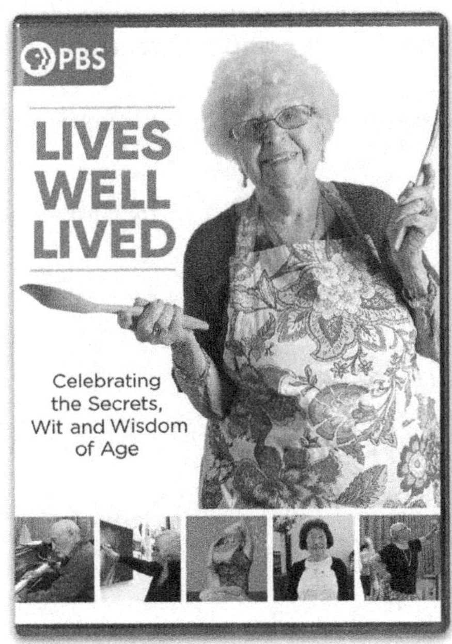

PLEASE REVIEW THIS BOOK!

Reviews help authors more than you might think. If you enjoyed *Lives Well Lived – Generations*, please consider leaving a review at your Amazon or regular bookstore—it would be greatly appreciated and help inspire more intergenerational readers!

...please share our project with your friends...

THANK YOU FOR YOUR SUPPORT!

FOLLOW US

For more information or to connect with Sky Bergman:

skybergmanproductions.com

lwlgenerations.com